Empowering Midwives and Obstetric Nurses

Edited by Amita Ray

Published in London, United Kingdom

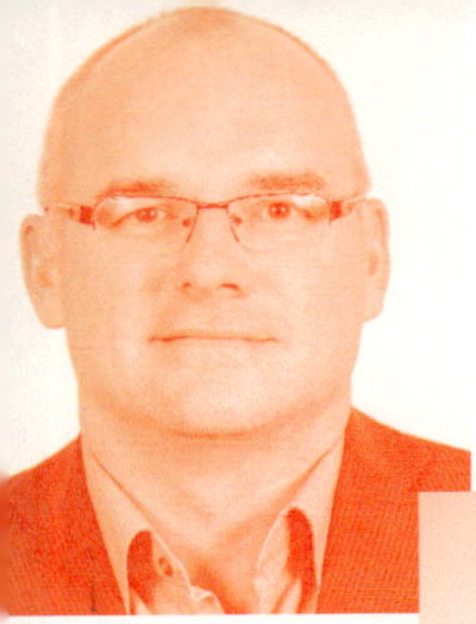
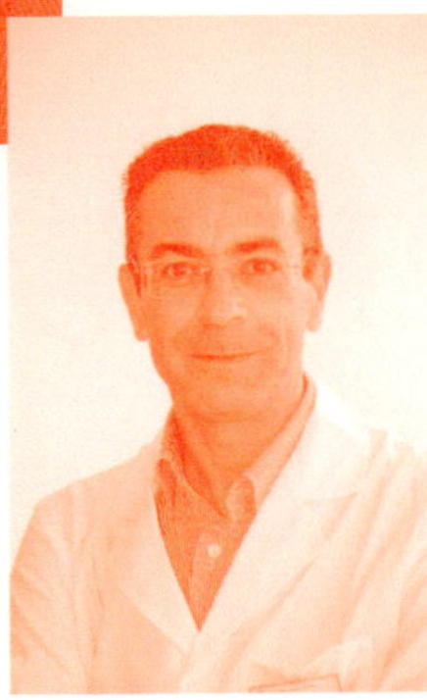
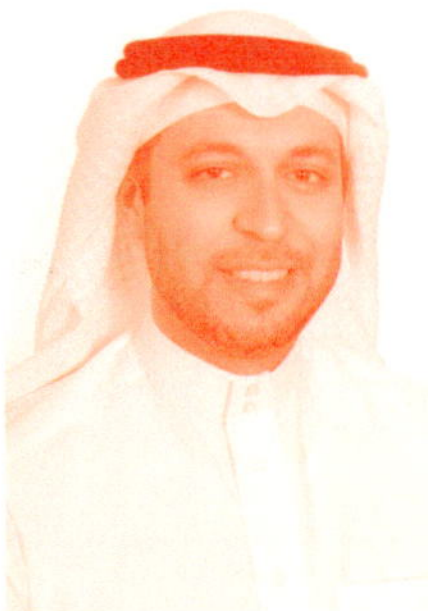
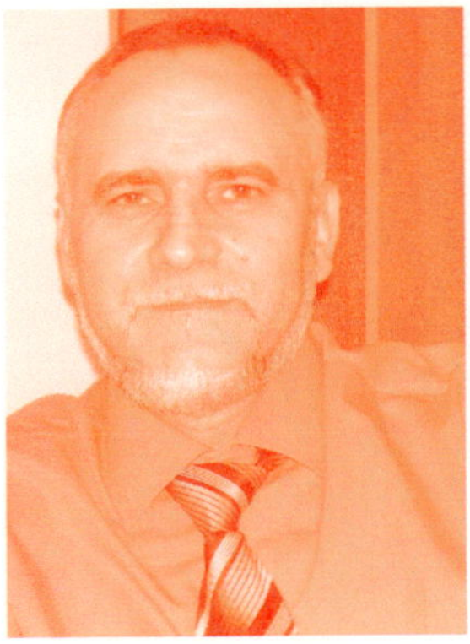
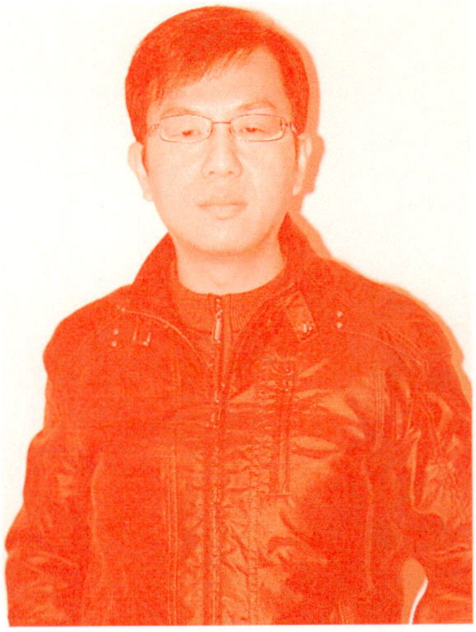
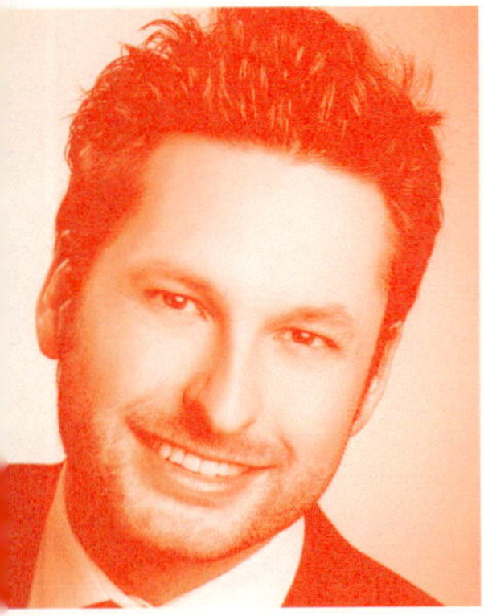
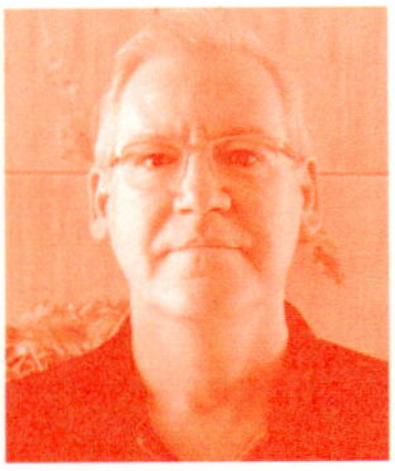

IntechOpen

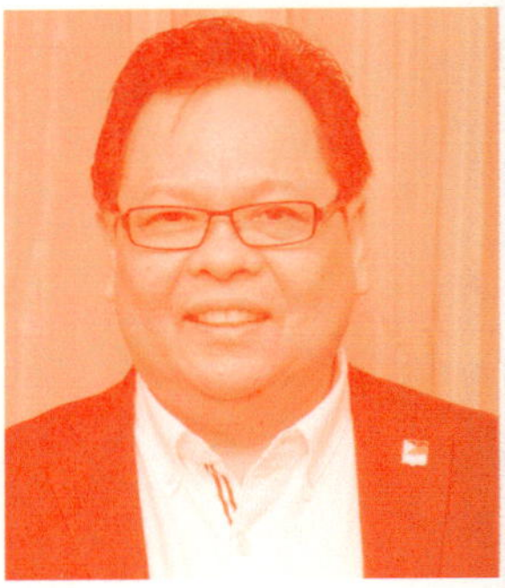
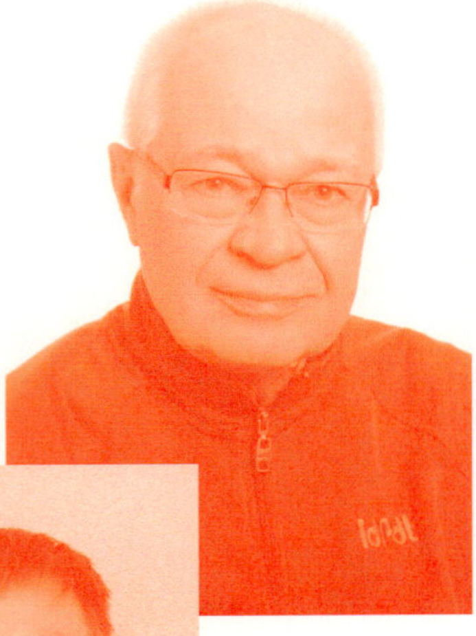
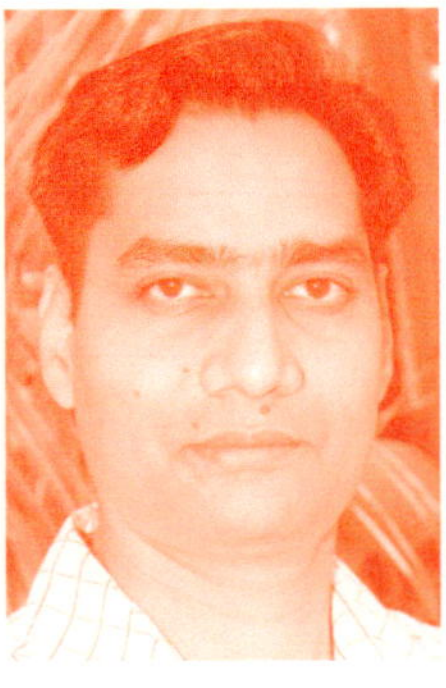
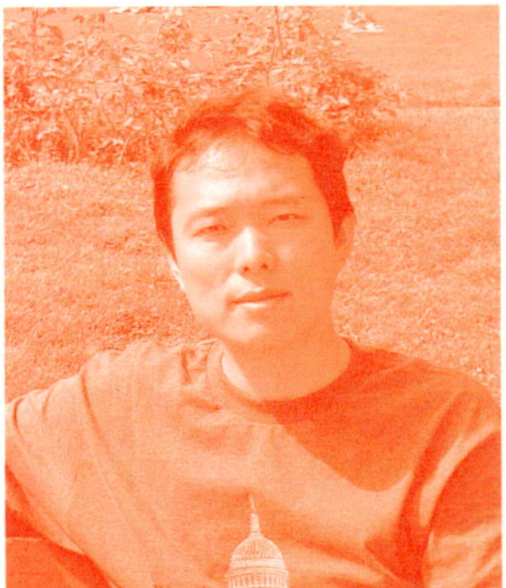
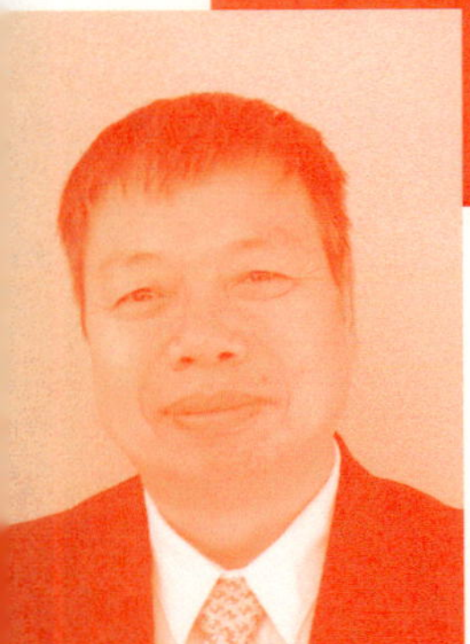
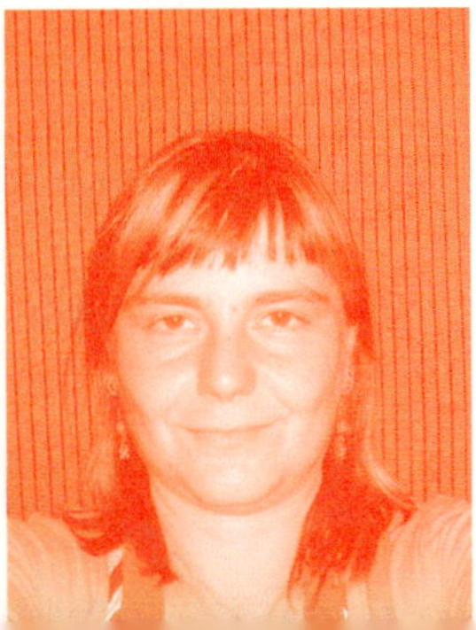

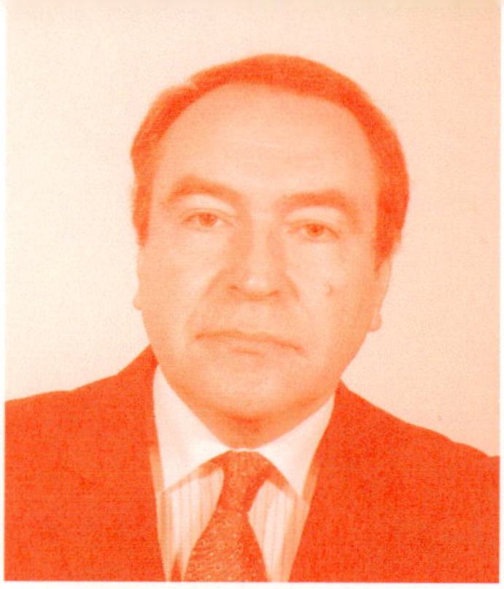

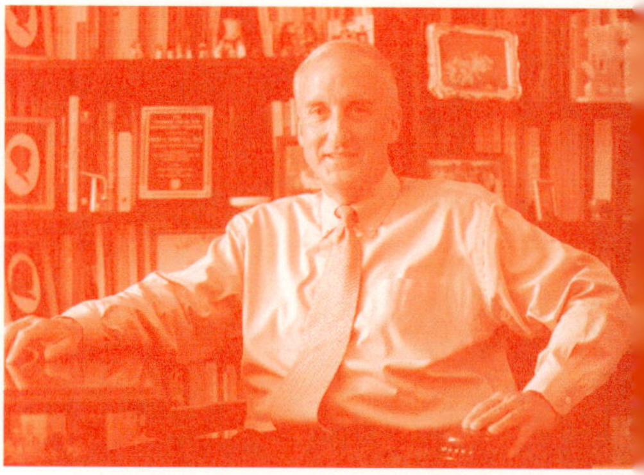

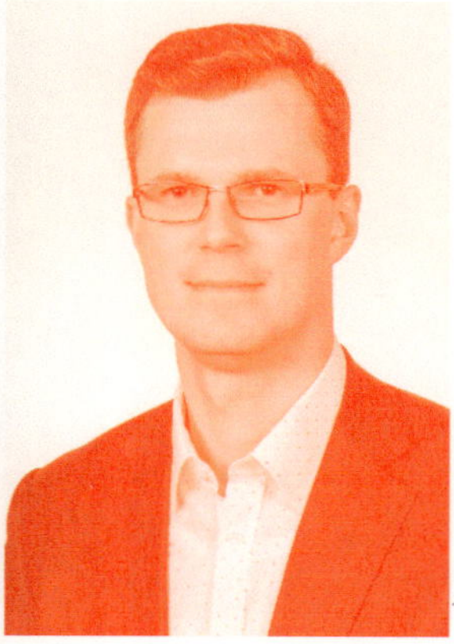

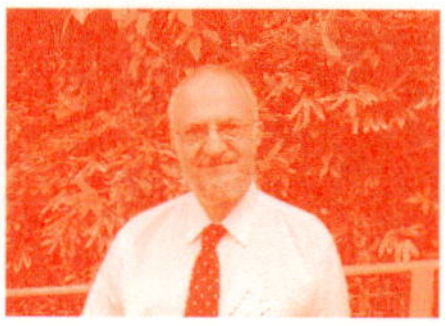

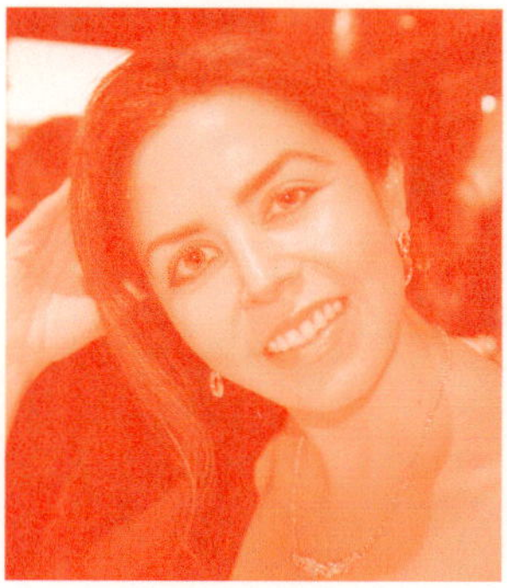

Supporting open minds since 2005

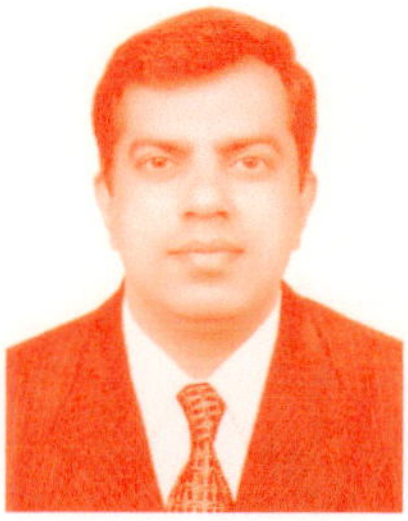

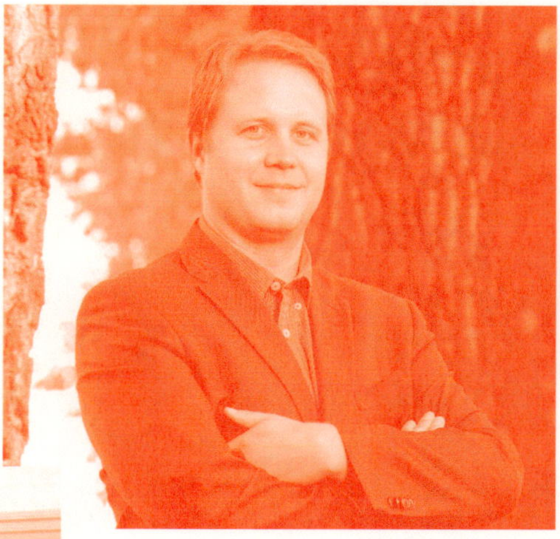

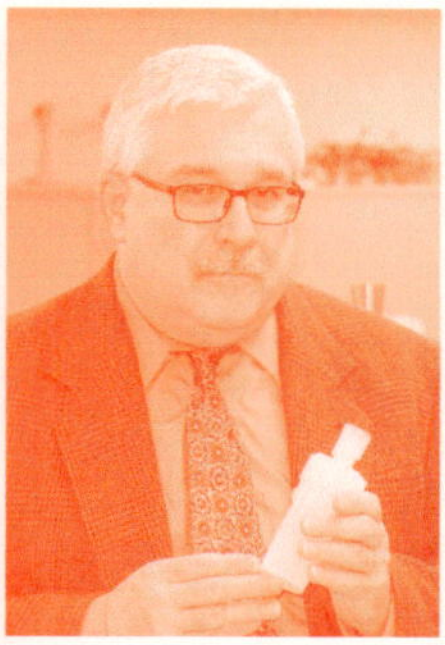

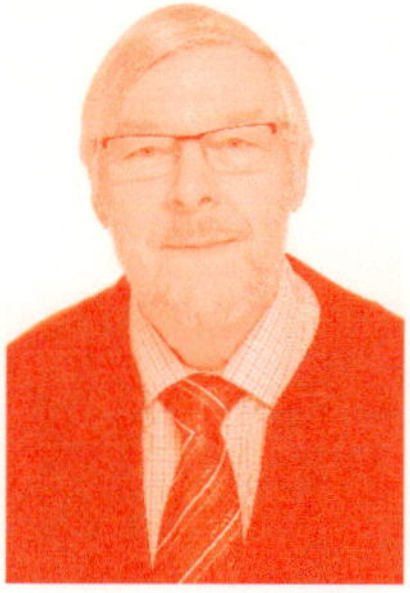

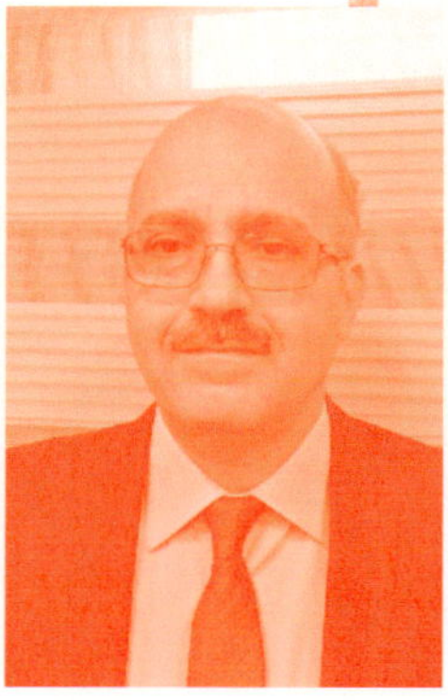

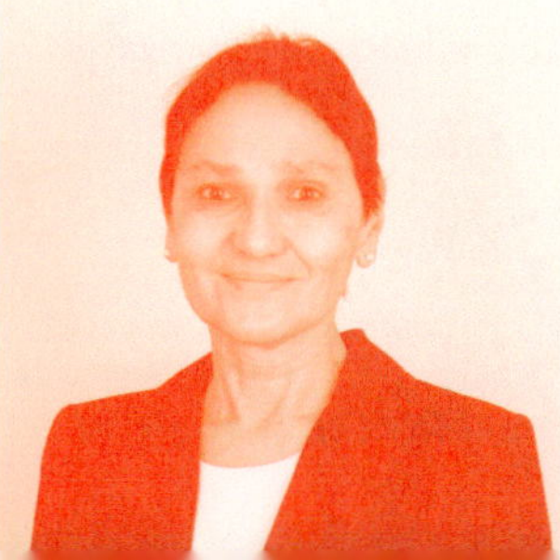

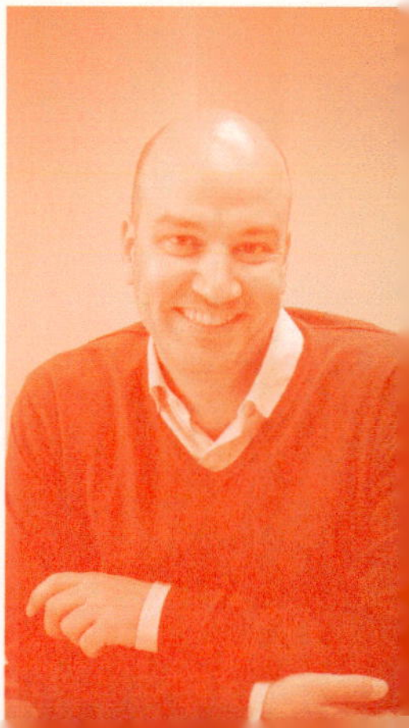

Empowering Midwives and Obstetric Nurses
http://dx.doi.org/10.5772/intechopen.78934
Edited by Amita Ray

Contributors
Jasneet Kaur, Suresh Ray, Maged Shendy, Hend Hindawy, Ibrahim Alatwi, Abdurhman Alatwi, Amr Salem, Teketel Ermias Geltore, Dereje Laloto Anore, Melash Belachew Asresie, Gizachew Worku Dagnew, Estela Arcos Griffiths, Ni Komang Yuni Rahyani Rahyani, Ni Made Dwi Mahayati, Made Widhi Gunapria Darmapatni, Ni Wayan Armini, Subrat Panda, Arindam Mallik, Ananya Das, Surajit Ray Baruah, Eugen Ancuta, Dragos Valentin Crauciuc, Dumitru Sofroni, Larisa Sfroni, Anton Emil, Carmen Anton, Eduard Crauciuc, Mihailov Claudia, Codrina Ancuta, Erhuvwukorotu Kollie, Kizito Omona, Callen Onyambu, Norah Tharamba, Amita Ray

First published in London, United Kingdom, 2021 by IntechOpen
IntechOpen is the global imprint of INTECHOPEN LIMITED, registered in England and Wales, registration number: 11086078, 5 Princes Gate Court, London, SW7 2QJ, United Kingdom
Printed in Croatia

British Library Cataloguing-in-Publication Data
A catalogue record for this book is available from the British Library

Additional hard and PDF copies can be obtained from orders@intechopen.com

Empowering Midwives and Obstetric Nurses
Edited by Amita Ray
p. cm.
Print ISBN 978-1-83969-065-5
Online ISBN 978-1-83969-066-2
eBook (PDF) ISBN 978-1-83969-067-9

Meet the editor

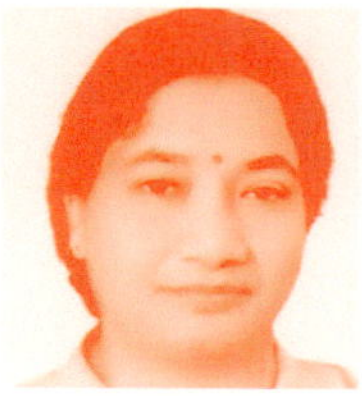

Prof. Dr. Amita Ray MBBS, MS, has worked as a clinician and medical teacher in various medical colleges all over India for the past thirty years. She has a master's degree in Obstetrics and Gynecology. She held a fellowship in Urogynecology and Gynae-Oncology at the Royal Adelaide Hospital, South Australia, and a fellowship in High-Risk Pregnancy Management at the Royal Oman Hospital, Sultan Quaboos University, Oman. She is passionate about her work among underprivileged women with pregnancy complications in tribal and rural areas. Dr. Ray is equally passionate about medical education. She completed a master's in Health Professionals Education and is a teaching faculty at a medical college. She has guided several post-graduate dissertations and introduced several innovative projects in health education, which have improved medical teacher efficiency in resource-constrained settings as a part of her Foundation for Advancement of Medical Education and Research (FAIMER) Fellowship. She has several publications in reputed national and international journals including British, American, and South Asian journals of obstetrics and gynecology. She has authored and co-authored several book chapters in obstetrics and gynecology textbooks used as a part of undergraduate and postgraduate education in India. She is passionate about evidence-based medicine and is an active member of different Cochrane Groups. She has authored and co-authored Cochrane Reviews for the Cochrane Pregnancy and Childbirth Group, Cochrane Cystic Fibrosis Group, and Cochrane Infectious Diseases Group. Dr. Ray is currently a professor in the Department of Obstetrics and Gynecology, IQ City Medical College, Durgapur, West Bengal, India. She is also the vice-principal and medical superintendent of the same institution.

Contents

Preface

This book is a collection of knowledge from experts in the health of pregnant mothers and their newborns. It deals with the art and science of the profession of midwifery, focusing on contemporary issues in midwifery including essential changes that have come about due to the COVID pandemic. It also deals with issues of domestic violence towards pregnant women.

This book supports learning and prepares readers for the challenges faced in contemporary midwifery healthcare. It presents 'must-have' information concerning both the theoretical and practical aspects of what it means to be a midwife. With extensive full-colour illustrations throughout, as well as activities and scenarios, this user-friendly textbook will support learners throughout their entire education programme. *Empowering Midwives and Obstetric Nurses* is essential reading for all pre-registration student midwives as well as newly qualified midwives. It is a practical approach to understanding the health of women and newborns.

Women in our society are becoming empowered to make informed and responsible choices regarding their health, but to do so they need the advocacy and support of nurses who care for them. This textbook focuses on women throughout their lifespan and arms the student or practicing nurse with essential information to care for women and their families, to assist them to make the right choices safely, intelligently, and with confidence.

Amita Ray
Department of Obstetrics and Gynecology,
IQ City Medical College,
Durgapur, West Bengal, India

Section 1

Introduction

Chapter 1

Introductory Chapter: Empowering Midwives and Obstetric Nurses

Amita Ray

1. Revising the old

The term midwifery has been coined from two Old English words "mid "which means with and "wif" which comes from woman. Taken together the word midwife means a person who is with the woman. This person could belong to any gender provided the person is with the woman during pregnancy as well as the whole process of childbirth and thereafter: probably the most eventful and crucial part of a woman's life.

Another word, more recently coined, is obstetrical nursing which in principles and domains follows the same as those of midwifery. Both midwifery and obstetrical nursing deal with knowledge and skills required for the nursing care of all normal and high risk pregnant woman during pregnancy, labor and after labor irrespective of the settings This discipline also includes the management of neonates and participation in family welfare programmes.

It is therefore not difficult to understand the importance of this discipline and appreciate the role of midwives in safeguarding woman's health. "The greatest privilege of human life is to become a midwife to the Awakening of the soul in another person" is how Plato defines the profession of midwifery. Their understanding and quick action at the time of childbirth plays a pivotal role in the health of the mother and the neonate and this job of midwives has been present since prehistoric times, long before other disciplines and professions evolved [1].

The profession of midwifery has cultural significance in almost all regions of the world. "In All Cultures, the Midwife's Place is on the Threshold of Life, Where Intense Human Emotions, Fear, Hope, Longing, Triumph, and Incredible Physical Power-Enable a New Human Being to Emerge. Her Vocation Is Unique." – Sheila Kitzinger. Only a few men specialized in the field in earlier times making it exclusively a woman's profession. In developing countries, there is a dearth of midwives added to this is the fact that they do not get enough support and are underpaid [2].

Women who specialize in midwifery have quite a lot of experience in the field. While the popularity of midwives reduced in the past two centuries, it has once again started rising with a lot of women preferring to give birth at home [2]. "It's not the making of babies, but the making of mothers that midwives see as the Miracle of Birth." – Barbara Katz Rothman.

2. Reinforcing the new

COVID has posed new challenges to the profession of midwifery. The pandemic has resulted in pregnant women and new mothers undergoing uncertainty and

IntechOpen

chaos particularly during this important phase of their lives. Providing evidence based and appropriate health care in such times has been more difficult for obstetricians, midwives and obstetric nurses [3]. In fact it has been a challenge for health care professionals to be mentally and physically healthy themselves.

This book aims to highlight certain important aspects of midwifery.It does not claim to cover all dimensions of the profession.Over the years and as is true for other disciplines and professions newer dimensions have been added to this profession as well.This book aims to highlight some old and some new dimensions of midwifery.

Author details

Amita Ray
Department of Obstetrics and Gynecology, IQ City Medical College, Durgapur, West Bengal, India

*Address all correspondence to: amitarays@gmail.com

References

[1] Dahlberg U'Aune I The woman's birth experience—The effect of interpersonal relationships and continuity of care Midwifery Volume 29, Issue 4, 2013, Pages 407-415

[2] 6138Noelyn Perriman, Deborah Lee Davis, Sally Ferguson What women value in the midwifery continuity of care model: A systematic review with meta-synthesis, Midwifery, Volume 62, 2018,Pages 220-229, ISSN 0266-6138

[3] Ollivier R ' Aston M, Price S, Dr. Sim M, Benoit B, Joy P, Iduye D, Nassaji N A, Mental Health & Parental Concerns during COVID-19: The Experiences of New Mothers Amidst Social Isolation, Midwifery, Volume 94, 2021,102902,ISSN 0266-

Section 2

Midwives in the Labor Room

Chapter 2

Vaginal Delivery

Kizito Omona

Abstract

Vaginal delivery refers to the birth of offspring in mammals or babies in humans, through the vagina, also known as the "birth canal". It is the natural method of birth for most mammals excluding those which lay eggs. For women who deliver vaginally, childbirth progresses in three stages: labor, delivery of the baby and delivery of the placenta. There are two types of vaginal delivery: Unassisted vaginal delivery and assisted vaginal delivery. In the later, this assistance can vary from use of medicines to emergency delivery procedures. The following types of vaginal delivery have been noted; (a) Spontaneous vaginal delivery (SVD) (b) Assisted vaginal delivery (AVD), also called instrumental vaginal delivery (c) Induced vaginal delivery and (d) Normal vaginal delivery (NVD), usually used in statistics or studies to contrast with a delivery by cesarean section. Delivery of a full-term newborn occurs at a gestational age of 37–42 weeks, usually determined by the last menstrual period or ultrasonographic dating and evaluation. Nearly 80% of newborns are delivered at full term while approximately 10% of singleton pregnancies are delivered preterm and 10% of all deliveries are post-term.

Keywords: cervical dilatation, uterine contraction, episiotomy, placental delivery

1. Introduction: Definitions - vaginal delivery

Vaginal delivery is defined as a natural birth process which does not usually require significant medical intervention [1]. It is the birth of offspring in mammals or babies in humans, through the vagina, also known as the "birth canal". Improvement of normal vaginal delivery can be made through proper management of normal labour, guided by current knowledge [1]. Most women deliver vaginally although the percentage of operative deliveries has increased from 21 percent in 1996 to 30 percent in 2005 respectively [1]. In the year 2013, out of the nearly four million births in the United States, there were approximately three million were vaginal deliveries [2]. In Australia in 2009, 70 percent of women delivered vaginally, of which 58.1% had spontaneous vaginal delivery [3]. In anticipating complications and preparing for vaginal delivery, accurate pregnancy dating is very essential [1]. There are relatively few absolute contraindications to vaginal delivery, meaning that most women deliver vaginally.

Most health experts, including World Health Organization (WHO), do recommend vaginal delivery for women whose babies have reached full term. In comparison to other methods of childbirth, vaginal delivery is the simplest process of delivery [4].

2. Types of vaginal delivery

There are different types of vaginal deliveries [5]; these are:

a. **Spontaneous vaginal delivery** (SVD) is one which occurs when a pregnant woman goes into labor without the use of drugs or other techniques to induce labor and she delivers her baby through the vagina (birth canal) without forceps, vacuum extraction or a cesarean section. Out of the about four million deliveries occurring in the United States each year, most of them are spontaneous vaginal deliveries. However, it should be noted that spontaneous vaginal deliveries are not advised for all mothers or pregnant women [4], as we shall see later. Of all women delivering in Australia in 2009, 58.1% had a spontaneous vaginal delivery [3].

b. **Assisted vaginal delivery** (AVD) also called **instrumental vaginal delivery or operative vaginal delivery** [6] occurs when a pregnant woman goes into labor, with or without the use of drugs or other techniques to induce labor and then delivers vaginally but with the use of special instruments such as forceps or a vacuum extractor. Assisted vaginal delivery is sometimes called operative vaginal delivery. Now days, assisted vaginal delivery is done in about 3% of vaginal deliveries in the United States [7]. Of all deliveries in Australia in 2009, 3.5% were delivered using forceps while 7.2% required vacuum extractions [3].

c. **Induced vaginal delivery** is a delivery which involves labor induction, where drugs or manual techniques are applied to initiate the process of labor.

d. **Normal vaginal delivery** (NVD) is a vaginal delivery, whether or not assisted or induced, usually used in statistics or studies to contrast with a delivery by cesarean section. In the year 2013, out of the nearly four million births in the United States, there were approximately three million were vaginal deliveries [2]. In Australia in 2009, 70 percent of women delivered vaginally [3].

3. Operative vaginal deliveries

3.1 Types of operative vaginal deliveries

As seen earlier (section 2b), Assisted vaginal delivery (AVD), also called instrumental vaginal delivery or operative vaginal delivery occurs when a pregnant woman goes into labor, with or without the use of drugs or other techniques to induce labor and then delivers vaginally but with the use of special instruments such as forceps or a vacuum extractor.

Henceforth, operative vaginal delivery involves application of forceps or a vacuum extractor to the fetal head to assist during the second stage of labour and facilitate delivery.

In United States of America (USA), assisted vaginal delivery is done in about 3% of all vaginal deliveries as per 2016 report of American College of Obstetricians and Gynecologists [6].

There are two main types of operative vaginal deliveries;

3.1.1 Vacuum extraction

Vacuum-assisted deliveries or vacuum extractions [6] involve attaching a soft cup, which has a handle, to the head of the baby when the baby is in the birth canal or vagina and a hand-held pump is then used to create suction that will help to facilitate delivery [5]. The doctor or midwife pulls the baby gently with each uterine contraction to facilitate delivery. In other words, a vacuum device is a suction-cup with a handle attached to it. This suction-cup is the one placed in the vagina and applied to the top of the baby's head. The doctor or midwife applies a gentle, well-controlled traction to help guide the baby out of the vagina as the mother keeps pushing with each uterine contraction [6].

The advantage of vacuum-assisted delivery is that this birth option has a lower risk than a Cesarean section in case of prolonged fetal distress.

However, the method carries the risks of minor scalp injuries or trauma and sometimes, bleeding of the scalp.

3.1.2 Forceps delivery

Forceps-assisted deliveries mean that curved instruments are to be used to facilitate delivery progress of the baby in the birth canal or vagina. Forceps which look like two large spoons are inserted into the vagina and are placed around the baby's head. They are then used to apply gentle traction to help guide the baby's head out of the vagina while the mother keeps pushing, with each uterine contraction [6]. Forceps delivery cannot be used if the baby is breech [5]. It can be an option if the mother is too tired or exhausted during pushing or if the baby has to be delivered more speedily than the naturally occurring process.

3.2 Pre-cautions for choice of operative vaginal delivery

The choice of devices used in operative vaginal delivery depends predominantly on the doctors or midwife's preference and experiences and these vary greatly. Operative vaginal deliveries are performed when the station of the fetal head is low, usually two centimeters below the maternal ischial spines [station +2] or lower than that. Minimal traction or rotation is then required to deliver the head [8].

Therefore, before starting an operative vaginal delivery, the doctor or midwife must do the following [9]:

- Confirm that cervical dilation is fully complete
- The doctor or midwife must confirm that there is engagement of fetal vertex at station +2 or lower
- Confirm that the membrane has ruptured
- The doctor or midwife must confirm that fetal position is very compatible with operative vaginal delivery
- Confirm that the maternal bladder is empty or else it must be drained
- Confirm that the maternal pelvis is adequate. This is done by clinically assessing the pelvic dimensions (clinical pelvimetry) in order to ascertain that the pelvis is adequate

The doctor or midwife need obtain informed consent, have adequate support and personnel as well as adequate analgesia or anesthesia. Neonatal care providers or nurses must have been alerted so that they can be ready to manage any neonatal complications that may arise. Anything less of the above requirements is very risky for operative vaginal delivery [9].

3.3 Indications for operative vaginal delivery

Basically, the indications for forceps delivery and vacuum extraction are the same [8]. They are [10];

- Prolonged second stage of labor, that is, from full cervical dilation to delivery of the fetus
- Suspicion of fetal compromise, such as abnormal heart rate pattern
- When there is need to shorten the second stage of labor for maternal benefit. This may be in the following circumstances; maternal cardiac dysfunction (such as left-to-right shunting), maternal exhaustion and neurologic disorders (such as spinal cord trauma). These conditions contraindicate pushing or prevent effective pushing.

3.4 Contraindications for operative vaginal delivery

Operative vaginal delivery is not permitted in some circumstances [8]. Contraindications include unengaged fetal head, unknown fetal position and certain fetal disorders such as hemophilia. In particular, Vacuum extraction is contraindicated in preterm pregnancies of less than 34 weeks of gestation. This is because risk of intra-ventricular hemorrhage is high [10].

3.5 Complications of operative vaginal delivery

Operative vaginal delivery poses some complications both to the mother and the baby [8]. The major complications are maternal injuries, fetal injuries and hemorrhage. These are common in particularly if the doctor or midwife is inexperienced or if the mother is not appropriately chosen. Significant maternal perineal trauma and neonatal bruising are more common with forceps delivery whereas shoulder dystocia, cephalohematoma, jaundice and retinal bleeding are more common with vacuum-assisted delivery.

4. Contraindications for vaginal delivery

Sometimes, vaginal deliveries may pose health risks for the mother, the baby or even both [4]. In such circumstances, medical experts recommend that pregnant women with the following conditions below must avoid spontaneous vaginal deliveries;

a. Mothers with complete placenta praevia. This is the situation where the baby's placenta fully covers the mother's cervix

b. Mothers with herpes virus having active lesions

c. Sometimes but not always, mothers with untreated HIV infection

d. Mothers who had more than one or two previous cesarean deliveries or uterine surgeries

In the circumstances above, the affected mothers are advised to deliver by Cesarean section. It's the desired alternative for mothers who have any one or more of those conditions.

5. Benefits and disadvantages of vaginal deliveries

5.1 Benefits

Vaginal delivery has the following benefits [5] to the mother and baby

a. Babies born vaginally tend to have fewer respiratory problems at birth and even afterwards.

b. The mother recovers much quicker than in other types of delivery, such as cesarean section.

c. Vaginal delivery has a lower rate of infection [11]. The baby will receive beneficial bacteria, that will help against infection [12]

d. A shorter hospital stay is realized in vaginal delivery than other delivery types, such as cesarean section. The recovery time is much faster in vaginal delivery [11]

e. The mother will be more likely to engage in early breastfeeding. A review of 53 international studies conducted in 2012 found that rates of early breastfeeding are lower after cesarean section than after vaginal delivery.

f. The mother will be less likely to have complications in future pregnancies

g. It is economically less costly compared to cesarean delivery. It has been argued that a Non-profit organization called 'FAIR Health' estimated that the average cesarean section in United States of America will cost about $16,907 whereas the average vaginal delivery costs nearly 30 percent less [11]

5.2 Disadvantages

Vaginal deliveries have the following disadvantages [5];

a. It carries higher risk of perineal tearing of the perineum.

b. Sometimes, a vaginal delivery may not be recommended in some medical conditions (see section 4 above).

6. Management of vaginal delivery

In order to manage normal vaginal delivery, many obstetric facilities tend to use a common labor suit, delivery, recovery and postpartum room. This is to allow the mother, the care giver and the neonate to remain in the same room throughout their stay. This makes it less costly. Some health facilities use a labor room and separate delivery suite, to which the mother is transferred when time for delivery comes. Usually, the mother's partner or any other support person is allowed in to give accompany to the mother [13]. In the delivery room, the perineum is washed and draped, and the neonate is delivered. After delivery, the woman may remain there or be transferred to a postpartum unit or section.

In managing normal vaginal delivery, the doctor or midwife must be well acquainted with the steps in conducting vaginal delivery [14]. See diagrammatic illustrations 1 and 2 below (**Figure 1**).

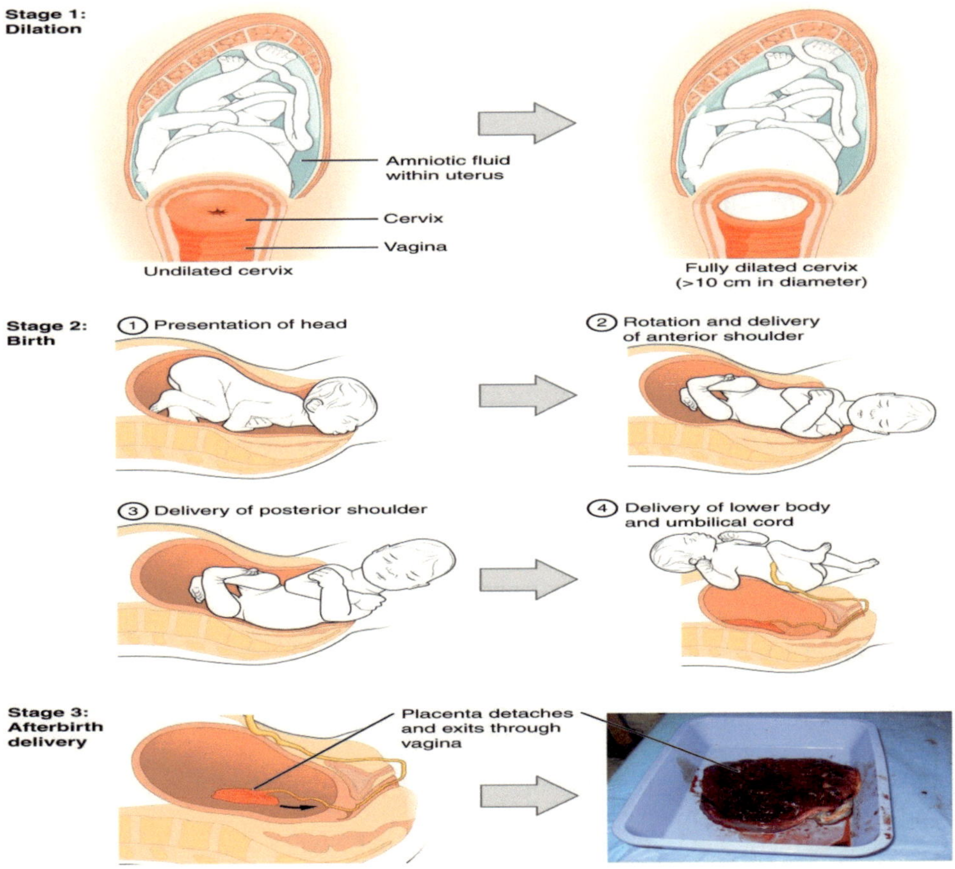

Figure 1.
Stages of vaginal delivery [15].

6.1 Anesthesia

There are many options for anesthesia. These are; local, regional and general anesthesia.

6.1.1 Local anesthesia

Usually, local anesthetics and opioids are frequently used. These medicines pass through the placenta and thus, before delivery, the medicine/drugs should be given in small doses to avoid toxicity in the neonate. The common toxicities related to local anaesthia are; central nervous system [CNS] depression and bradycardia [13].

It must be noted that opioids used alone do not provide adequate analgesia and so are most often used with anesthetics.

In the option for anesthesia, most of the local anesthetic methods used include; pudendal blocks and perineal infiltration as well as para-cervical blocks.

a. **Pudendal block:** Pudendal blocks are used rarely. Instead of this, epidural injections are more preferred. In this, a local anesthetic is injected through the vaginal wall so as to bathe the pudendal nerve as it crosses the ischial spine. In this way, the block anesthetizes the lower vagina, perineum and posterior vulva. However, the anterior vulva, innervated by lumbar dermatomes, is thus not anesthetized [13]. Usually, pudendal block is considered a safe and simple method for spontaneous vaginal deliveries if the delivery is uncomplicated. It is even more so especially if the mother wishes to bear down and push or when the labor is advanced such that there is no time for epidural injection. It should be noted that pudendal block may have some complications which include intravascular injection of anesthetics, hematoma and infections.

b. **Infiltration of the perineum**: Infiltration of the perineum with an anesthetic is commonly, even if the method is not as effective as a well-administered pudendal block.

c. **Para-cervical block:** This is rarely appropriate for delivery because incidence of fetal bradycardia is >10% [16]. It is used mainly for abortion in the first or early second trimester. The technique involves injecting 5 to 10 mL of 1% lidocaine or chloroprocaine, which has a shorter half-life. Injection is at the 3 and 9 o'clock positions. The analgesic response is usually short-lasting.

6.1.2 Regional anesthesia

There are several methods are available for regional anesthesia;

a. **Lumbar epidural injection:** Lumbar epidural injection of a local anesthetic is the most commonly preferred method. Epidural analgesia is being increasingly used for delivery, including in cesarean delivery. It has basically replaced pudendal and para-cervical blocks. Note that the drugs can be titrated as needed during the course of labor when epidural analgesia is used. Bupivacaine, the local anesthetics often used for epidural injection has a longer duration of action and slower onset than those used for pudendal block. In pudendal block, lidocaine is used, instead.

b. **Spinal injection:** Spinal injection into the para-spinal sub-arachnoid space may be used. However, this is predominantly for cesarean delivery but less often for vaginal deliveries. This is because it is short-lasting, preventing its use during labor, and it has a small risk of spinal headache afterward. Patients must be constantly attended to when spinal injections are used and vital signs must be monitored every 5 minutes to detect and treat possible hypotension.

6.1.3 General anesthesia

General anesthesia is not recommended for routine delivery because potent and volatile inhalation drugs, such as isoflurane, can cause marked depression in the fetus [16].

Again, on rarely basis, during vaginal delivery, 40% nitrous oxide, with oxygen can be used for analgesia. This is so, as long as verbal contact with the mother is well maintained [13].

However, for induction of general anesthesia during cesarean section, thiopental, which is a sedative-hypnotic, is predominantly given intravenously with other drugs such as; succinylcholine and nitrous oxide plus oxygen. When thiopental is used alone, it provides inadequate analgesia and yet with it (thiopental), induction is more rapid and recovery is very prompt. Thiopental may become concentrated in the fetal liver and this prevents its levels from becoming high in the central nervous system (CNS). High levels of thiopental in the CNS may cause neonatal depression, a situation very detrimental to desired outcome of delivery.

6.2 Analgesia

In other studies, analgesia is recommended [17]. In this case, an attempt with a peridural approach or with the use of short-acting narcotics is advisable. Platelet counts more than 50,000/mL for cesarean delivery, more than 20,000/mL for vaginal delivery, more than 75,000/mL for epidural anesthesia, and more than 50,000/mL for spinal anesthesia in that order are considered safe for delivery.

6.3 Delivery of the fetus

In order to fully comprehend the delivery of fetus, one needs to know the mechanism of labour well. It involves the passive movement the fetus must undertake in order to negotiate through the maternal bony pelvis. Thus labour can be broken down into the following respective stages; descent, engagement, neck flexion, internal rotation, crowning, extension of the presenting part, restitution, internal rotation and lateral flexion. The readers are advised to read other chapter of this book, where labour was discussed in details. Knowledge of pelvic anatomy and perimetry becomes vital, which is lacking in this section.

Thus, in delivering the fetus, a vaginal examination is done to ascertain the position and station of the fetal head. The head is usually the presenting part of the fetus, bu. rarely the buttock [13]. If effacement is completed and the cervix is fully dilated, then the mother is asked to bear down and strain with each uterine contraction. This helps to move the head through the pelvis and progressively dilate the vaginal introitus so that more and more of the head comes out. The moment about 3 or 4 cm of the head is visible during a uterine contraction in nulliparas, the following maneuvers can then facilitate vaginal delivery and reduce risk of perineal tear;

- The doctor or midwife, if he or she is right-handed, will place the left palm over the fetus's head during a contraction to control progress.
- Concurrently, the doctor or midwife should place his or her curved fingers of the right hand against the dilating perineum, through which the infant's brow or chin is felt. See **Figure 2** below.
- In order to advance the head, the doctor or midwife should wrap his or her hand in a towel and then with the curved fingers, he or she should apply pressure against the underside of the brow or chin. This maneuver is known as 'modified Ritgen's maneuver' [13].

An **episiotomy** many be performed as necessary. However, episiotomy is not commonly desired for most normal vaginal deliveries. It should be considered only and only if the perineum does not stretch adequately, so that it is obstructing delivery of the baby. In this case, consider infiltrating a local anesthetic if epidural analgesia seems inadequate. Episiotomy relieves excessive stretching and possible irregular tear of the perineal tissues, including anterior tears, which could ensue in it absence. The recommended episiotomy incision which should be preferred is one that extends only through the skin and perineal body without disrupting the anal sphincter muscles (2nd -degree episiotomy). This is because it is easier to repair than a perineal tear. See **Figure 3** below for possible sites of episiotomy.

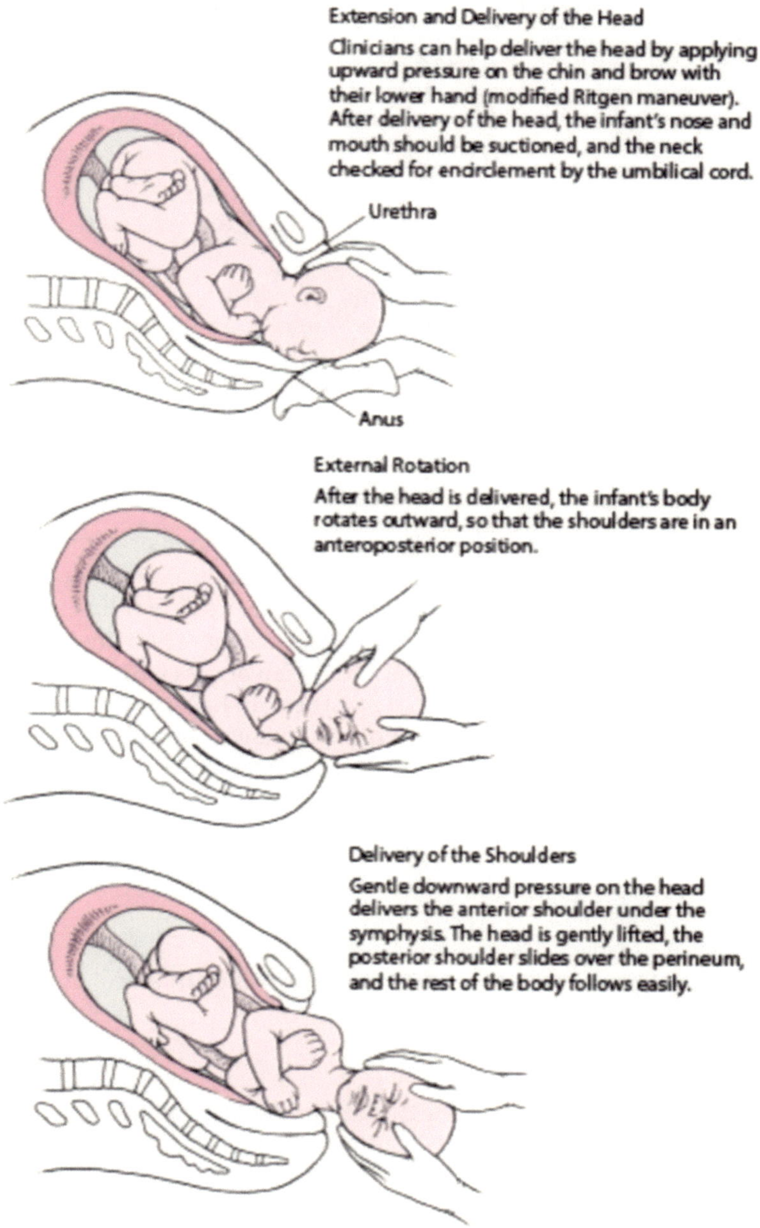

Figure 2.
Steps in conducting vaginal delivery [13].

6.4 Delivery of the placenta

It is common knowledge that active management of the 3rd stage of labour reduces the risk of postpartum hemorrhage. Active management of 3rd stage of labour includes giving the mother a uterotonic drug such as oxytocin as immediate as the fetus is delivered. This uterotonic drug helps the uterus to contract effectively and decrease bleeding due to uterine atony.

Oxytocin, given as 10 units intramuscularly or infusion of 20 units/1000 mL of normal saline at 125 mL/hour is considered. It should not be given as an intravenous bolus in order to minimize the risk of cardiac arrhythmia which might otherwise occur.

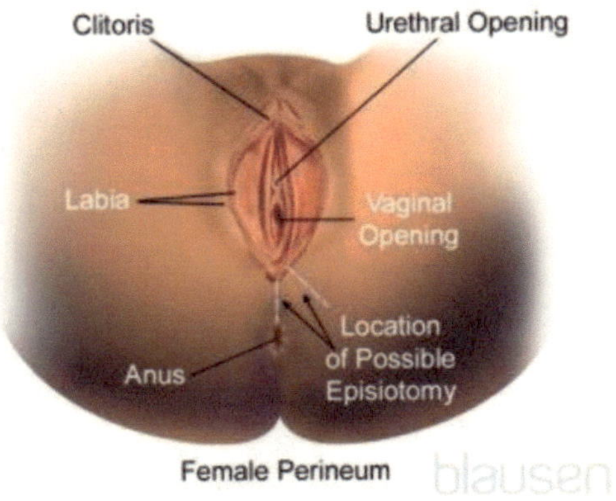

Figure 3.
Possible sites of episiotomy in vaginal delivery [13].

Upon successful delivery of the baby and administration of oxytocin, the doctor or midwife should gently and controllably pull the cord and place his or her hand gently on the mother's abdomen over the uterine fundus. This is to detect contractions [13]. Note that separation of placenta from uterus usually occurs during the 1st or 2nd contraction. This often occurs with a gush of blood from behind the separating placenta. The mother can help to deliver the placenta by bearing down. In case the mother cannot bear down and substantial bleeding occurs, the placenta should be evacuated by the doctor or midwife placing his or her hand on the abdomen and then exerting firm downward (caudal) pressure on the uterus. This kind of procedure must be done only on condition that the uterus feels firm, otherwise, pressure on a flaccid uterus can cause the uterus to invert, thus worsening the problem.

7. The Do's and Don'ts when conducting vaginal delivery

7.1 The Do's

For successful vaginal delivery, the doctor or midwife may have to consider the following things to be done;

- Be prepared and knowledgeable on conduction of vaginal delivery and equipments to use
- Seek consent for vaginal delivery from the mother or next-of-kin
- Allay mother's anxiety
- Wait for labour to progress spontaneously, while monitoring contraction, cervical dilation, fetal descent and heart rate
- Have your equipments, also called delivery set, placed at the proper position in labour suit near the mother
- Have your oxytocics ready and placed in proper position
- Put on your sterile gloves

- Do attentive waiting on the mother
- Conduct vaginal delivery as labour progresses and the baby comes out
- Call for help where appropriate
- Have neonatal resuscitation equipments ready and functional

7.2 The Don'ts

- In vaginal delivery, take care that you do not do the following;
- Do not fail to seek consent for delivery from the mother or next-of-kin
- Do not fear to call for help whenever it is required
- Do not use unsterile equipments
- Do not conduct vaginal delivery without ascertaining the availability of an assistant or a senior midwife or doctor
- Do not conduct vaginal delivery without preparing your delivery set
- Do not conduct vaginal delivery without ascertaining the availability of oxytocics
- Do not conduct vaginal delivery without ascertaining availability neonatal resuscitation equipments
- Do not conduct vaginal delivery without ascertaining the functionality of your neonatal resuscitation equipments
- Do not be absent minded

8. Conclusion

For a full-term newborn, vaginal delivery means to deliver the baby at a gestational age of 37–42 weeks, from the mother's first day of the last menstrual period. This is determined by an accurate history taking from the mother or by ultrasonographic dating and evaluation. Some mothers, for one reason or another, may not adequately know their first day of the last normal menstrual period. In this case, reliance on history from the mother may be misleading. However, the Naegel rule is the use of a commonly known formula to predict the expected date of devilery. The formula is based on the date of the first day of the last normal menstrual period of the mother. The rule assumes a menstrual cycle of 28 days and mid-cycle ovulation, at 14 day from the first normal menstrual day. This means that the formula may not be applicable for women whose cycles are either less than 28 days or more than 28 days and whose ovulation may occur before or after day 14. In this case, however, ultrasonographic dating can be much more accurate, especially if it is done in early pregnancy, before 12 weeks of gestation. Ultrasonographic dating done earlier than 12 weeks are more accurate than those done at 12 weeks or above 12 weeks. Again, this might depend on the level of experience and knowledge of the user of the ultrasound machine. Vaginally, approximately 11% of singleton pregnancies are delivered preterm whereas 10% of all deliveries are post-term. Good knowledge of normal vaginal deliveries thus, forms the basis for management of complicated deliveries.

Acknowledgements

I do acknowledge the technical guidance of my colleagues in the Faculty of Health Sciences of Uganda Martyrs University. In a special way I appreciate Ms. Scovia Mbabazi, the former Associate Dean of the faculty.

Conflict of interest

The author declares no conflict of interest.

Author details

Kizito Omona
Uganda Martyrs University, Faculty of Health Sciences, Kampala, Uganda

*Address all correspondence to: kizitoomona@gmail.com; komona@umu.ac.ug

References

[1] **PATTERSON, D. A., WINSLOW, M. and MATUS, C. D.** Spontaneous Vaginal Delivery. 2008. Vol. 78, 3, pp. 336-341. Available at:https://www.aafp.org/afp/2008/0801/p336.html.

[2] **Martin, J. A., et al.** Births: final data for 2013. 2015. Vol. 64, 1, pp. 1-65. Available at: https://www.cdc.gov/nchs/data/nvsr/nvsr64/nvsr64_01.pdf.

[3] **Healthengine.** Vaginal Delivery. *healthengine.com.* [Online] 2009. https://healthengine.com.au/info/vaginal-delivery#c1.

[4] **Cirino, E.** Spontaneous Vaginal Delivery. *Healthline.org.* [Online] 2017. https://www.healthline.com/health/pregnancy/spontaneous-vaginal-delivery.

[5] **Oberg, E. N. D.** 7 Childbirth Delivery Methods and Types. *Medicinenet.com.* [Online] n.d. https://www.medicinenet.com/7_childbirth_and_delivery_methods/article.htm.

[6] **American College of Obsterics and Gynaecology.** Assisted Vaginal Delivery. *acog.org.* [Online] 2016. https://www.acog.org/womens-health/faqs/assisted-vaginal-delivery.

[7] **American College of Obstetricians and Gynacologists.** Assisted Vaginal Delivery | ACOG. *acog.org.* [Online] n.d. https://www.acog.org/search#q=Vaginal%20Deliveries&sort=relevancy.

[8] **Moldenhauer, J. S.** Operative Vaginal Delivery. *msdmanuals.com.* [Online] 2020. https://www.msdmanuals.com/professional/gynecology-and-obstetrics/abnormalities-and-complications-of-labor-and-delivery/operative-vaginal-delivery.

[9] **Royal College of Obstetricians and Gynaecologists.** *Operative Vaginal Delivery.* London : Royal College of Obstetricians and Gynaecologists, 2011.

[10] **Cargill, Y. M., et al.** Guidelines for operative vaginal birth. 2004. Vol. 26, 8, pp. 747-761. DOI: 10.1016/s1701-2163(16)30647-8.

[11] **ROGERS-ANDERSON, S.** VAGINAL BIRTH BENEFITS FOR BABY & MOTHER. *thetot.com.* [Online] 2020. https://www.thetot.com/pregnancy-and-fertility/9-benefits-of-a-vaginal-birth/.

[12] **Iara, M. L., et al.** Chapter 11 - The Human Vaginal Microbiome. [book auth.] J. Faintuch and S. Faintuch. *Microbiome and Metabolome in Diagnosis, Therapy, and other Strategic Applications.* NY : Academic Press, 2019, 11, pp. 109-114.

[13] **Artal-Mittelmark, R.** Management of Normal Delivery. *msdmanuals.com.* [Online] 2019. https://www.msdmanuals.com/professional/gynecology-and-obstetrics/normal-labor-and-delivery/management-of-normal-delivery.

[14] **Pillitteri, A.** "Chapter 15: Nursing Care of a Family During Labor and Birth". *Maternal & Child Health Nursing: Care of the Childbearing & Childrearing Family.* Maryland : Lippincott Williams, 2010, 15.

[15] **Wikipedia.** Child Birth. *en.wikipedia.org.* [Online] 2020. https://en.wikipedia.org/wiki/Childbirth.

[16] **LeFevre, M. L.** Fetal heart rate pattern and postparacervical fetal bradycardia. 1984. Vol. 64, 3, pp. 343-346. PMID: 6462564.

[17] **Benson, A. and Oren, R.** 54 - The Liver in Pregnancy. [book auth.] J. S. Arun, et al. *Zakim and Boyer's Hepatology (Seventh Edition).* NY : Elsevier, 2018.

Chapter 3

Preterm Labour

Maged Shendy, Hend Hendawy, Amr Salem,
Ibrahim Alatwi and Abdurahman Alatawi

Abstract

Preterm delivery is defined as delivery before 37 weeks completed gestation. It represents a major cause of neonatal morbidity and mortality and accounts for 5–10% of all deliveries. Cervical length assessment between 16–24 weeks and positive fetal fibronectin beyond 21 weeks gestation are proved to useful tools in prediction of preterm labour. Treating asymptomatic bacteruia and bacterial vaginosis in high-risk women reduces the incidence of preterm labour. Cervical cerclage is recommended to reduce the incidence of preterm birth in women with 2nd trimester losses and those with cervical length of 25 mm or less on transvaginal ultrasound between 16–24 weks gestation. Atosiban and nifidipine are currently the agents of choice in tocolysis. Antenal steriods in womens with threating preterm labour reduces the perinatal morbidties. Magnisum sulphate role is established for neuroprotection especially in extreme gestations between 24–30 weeks. Vaginal delivery is mode of choice for delivery with consideration to avoid fetal blood sampling, fetal scalp electrodes and ventouse prior to 34 weeks gestations. Caesarean section is considered for obstetric reasons that guide labour management at term.

Keywords: definition, maternal morbidity, feral morbidity, risk factors, tocolysis, antenatal steroids

1. Introduction

Preterm delivery is defined as delivery before 37 weeks completed gestation. It represents a major cause of neonatal morbidity and mortality in both developed and developing countries with European and North American figures ranges between 5–10% of all deliveries. In the UK it represents 7.3% of live births

Extreme preterm birth is defined as preterm birth prior to 28 weeks gestation. It accounts for 5–10% of preterm deliveries. The major concern of extreme preterm birth is the significant risk of neonatal mortality as the survival rates are very low at these gestations (0.4% at 22 weeks, 7% at 24 weeks) while the main concern of preterm births above 28 weeks is the neonatal morbidity as the survival rates are 77% at 28 weeks and 97% at 36 weeks.

2. Aetiology

The aetiology of preterm labour is multifactorial with a common pathway reslutting in increased relasee of prostaglandins and cytokines within the cervix, myometrium and fetal membranes. The release of prostaglandins is triggered by infective or inflammatory process [1], uterine overdistension as in cases with polyhydraminons and mutiple preganacy or choriodecudidual haemorrhage as in cases with abruption.

In modern obstetrics, 30–40% of preterm deliveries are iatrogenic. The most common cause of which is severe pre-eclampsia associated with intrauterine growth restriction (IUGR) and antenatal fetal distress. Other common iatrogenic preterm deliveries include, Grade 3 and 4 placenta praevia or placenta abruption with major bleeding, sever IUGR with absent or reversed end-diastolic flow. It is also notable that the increased number of large loop excision of transformation zone (LLETZ) procedures for abnormal cervical cells leads to cervical scarring and iatrogenic cervical incompetence and hence preterm delivery.

3. Prediction of preterm labour

Identifying high risk patients is crucial in managing and preventing preterm labour. Prediction of preterm labour is possble through; risk assessment, uterine activity monitoring, cervical length assessment and fetal fibronectin assessment.

3.1 History taking and risk assessment

Patients with previous preterm labour are at higher risk of having pretem term birth. The risk is 17% after one previous preterm delivery and increases to 28% after two preterm deliveries. Patients with previous preterm premature rupture of membranes (PROM) [2], previous second trimester loss and thoese who are known to have cervical incomptence and congenital uterine anaomalies are at higher risk for preterm birth. Fruther more uterine overdistention as with Polyhydraminos and mutiple pregnancy is associated with preterm delivery. Patient with placental abruption are also known to be at higher risk of preterm labour.

Scoring systems were developed in attempts to achieve accurate and numerical score to help the management of preterm labour. However; the scoring systems proved to have poor sensitivity and poor postive predictive values as more that 50% of preterm labour occurs in the first pregnancy and in womens with no risk factors [3].

3.2 Monitoring uterine activity

It notable that uterine activity increases prior to onset of pretrm labour by 24 hours. However, the use of home uterine contraction monitors or self palpations has not proven to be useful as they had poor postive predictive vlaues and their use did not improve the perinatal outcomes.

3.3 Assessment of cervical length

Clinical assessment of cervical status in terms of dilatation, softening and effacement can predict preterm labour, However it has low sensitivity and repeated vaginal examination in it self may incease the cervical prostaglandins relase and subsquently increase the incidnce of preterm labour.

Utrasound assessment of cervical length is a reliable method and highest predictive value up to 70% is notable with cervical length under 25 mm in womens with risk factors for preterm labour. Serial cervical length assessment is recommended in hight isk group between 16–24 weeks. Cervical length is best measured by transvaginal scan with empty bladder as full bladder may lead to false increase in the cervical length measurments. The risk of preterm labour increases from 1% at cervical length of 25 mm to 4% at 15 mm cervical length. The marked increased risk is notable at 5 mm cervical length with preterm birth risk of 78% [4, 5].

Cervical length assessment is not routine in womens with no risk factors for preterm birth as the positive predictive value is low in this group. Also, preventive interventions as cervical cerclage is not recommended in low risk group as they have shown no improvement in the outcome in this group [4].

The presence of funnelling of the internal os is another helpful finding in predicting the preterm birth, However, it is less accurate compared to cervical length assessment due to inter and intra observer variations [6].

3.4 Fetal fibronectin testing

Fetal fibronectin is normally present in high concentration prior to 21 weeks of gestation in cervical and vaginal secretions prior to membranes fusion. Inflammatory process, uterine overdistension and choriodecidual haemorrhage increase fetal fibronectin secretion after 21 weeks gestation.

Fetal fibronectin testing by swabbing the posterior fornix or ectocervix between 22 and 34 weeks gestation in recommended as postive results in high risk group especially in presence of symptoms warrant admistration of steriods and hospital admission. Fetal fibronectin testing is not recommeded in womens with no risk factors as it has not shown to be effective in improving the outcome despite more than half of preterm birth occurs in this group [7].

Testing for fetal fibronectin is contraindicated before 22 weeks gestation, in presence of preterm premature rupture of membranes, active vaginal bleeding and intercourse in the previous 24 hours.

Other biochemical markers such as Insulin like growth factor binding protein-1, interleukin-6, interleukin-8 and tumour necrosis factor-alpha (TNF-α) were assessed in research setting for use in predicting preterm labour. However, none of those markers is currently used in routine practice [8].

4. Neonatal morbidity and mortality of preterm labour

Preterm birth is associated with significant neonatal morbidities such as respiratory distress syndrome, necrotizing enterocolitis, retinopathy of prematurity, neonatal sepsis, intraventricular haemorrhage and periventricular leucomalacia. Longterm impact of prematurity are mainly cognitive and motor impairement which are more prevelant in extreme preterm births. Prolongation of pregnancy with tocolytic agents and adminstration of antenatal steriods signficantly reduces the neonatal morbidities in preterm births [1, 9].

EPICure data [9] may be useful tool in counselling the parents about fetal prognosis. Neonatal mortality is higher with preterm birth at lower gestational ages with survival rate of 7% at 24 weeks compared to 77% at 28 weeks and 97% at 32 weeks. The survival rates improves 2.2% daily between 24 and 28 weeks gestions. Preterm delivery at 36 weeks is associated with 99% survival rate [1, 9, 10].

5. Prevention of preterm delivery

Mutiple preventive measures were tested for prevention of preterm labour such as treatment of asymptomatic bacteruria and bacterial vaginosis, prophylactic antibiotics in womens with postive fetal fibronectin and reduced cervical length, cervical cerclage, prophlactic tocolysis and hormonal supplements. Some were proved to be effective in reducing preterm deliveries while others shown no significant diffierence in the outcome regarding the incidance of preterm birth and its associated morbidities.

a. Bacterial vaginosis occurs in 10–22% of pregnant womens with unknown aetiology. Treating the bacterial vagnoisis and hence reducing its associated inflammatory process was proved to reduce the incidance of preterm birth in womens with risk factors for preterm labour especially those with postive fetal fibronectin testing. Asymptomatic bacteruria occurs in 2–9% pregnant womens and its associated inflammtory process can participate in increasing prostagladins levels in cervicovaginal secretions and hence the preterm birth. Treating asymptomatic bacteruria in high risk group reduces the incidence of preterm birth but not in low risk group.

b. Antibiotic treatment for prophylactic antibiotics in womens with postive fetal fibronectin and in womens reduced cervical length in absence of infective or inflammatory process is not recommeded due to limited evidence and lack of proven efficacy.

c. Cervical cerclage proved to reduce the incidence of preterm birth in women with 2nd trimester losses and those with cervical length of 25 mm or less on transvaginal ultrasound between 16–24 weks gestation [4, 11]. Cervical cerclage can be done by transvaginal route (McDonald or Shirodkar techniques) or transadominal route when there is insufficient cervical tissue to hold the suture or when the vaginal approach has failed previously [1, 4]. Counselling prior such procedure is essential to involve the pros and cons. Complications of the procedure can include; bleeding, infection (endometritis), increased frequency of contractions, cervical trauma, preterm premature rupture of membranes, suture displacement, sepsis, cervical scarring. Cervical cerclage is contraindicated in presence of fetal anomaly, intrauterine infection, active bleeding and preterm premature rupture of membranes [1, 6].

d. Prophylactic tocolysis for high risk women has not proved to reduce the preterm birth rate and is not recommended.

e. Progesterone supplement via vaginal or intramuscular route on weekly basis till 36 weeks can be considered to promote reduction of uterine activity. Its use is limited to clinical trials in European guidlines [12, 13] while the recent NICE guideline in UK and in North America, progesterone supplementation is recommended for clinical use for reuction of preterm births [1, 14].

f. Use of cervical pessaries, bed rest and restrticting physical activity and intercourse have no proved evidence of preventing preterm labour [15, 16].

6. Management of preterm labour

The mangement of preterm labour fall into five areas; the use of tocolysis, adminstration of antibiotics, admistration of antenatal steriods, magnisum sulphate for neuroprotection and finally the considerations for the mode of delivery.

7. Tocolysis

It is important to realise that the aim of tocolysis in modern obstertics is limited to gain few days to allow admistration of antenatal steriods which proved to reduce perinatal morbidities in preterm birth and allow in utero transfer (**Table 1**).

Tocolytics	Mechanism	Dose	Side effects	Contraindications
Ritodrine - b2-agonists Currently not in use	b2-receptor stimulation reduces free intra-cellular Ca^{+2} via cyclic AMP and hence muscle relaxation	50–100 μ g/ min IV then, increase by 50 μ g/min every 10 min. (up to 350 μ g/ min)	Maternal; Hyperglycemia hypokalemia Tremors and nervousness Dyspnea and chest pain Palpitations and arrhythmia Hypotension Pulmonary edema Fetal/neonatal; Tachycardia Hypoglycemia Hypocalcemia Hyperbilirubinemia hypotension IVH	Dysrhythmias or other significant cardiac disease Diabetes mellitus Uncontrolled thyroid disease
Calcium channel blockers (CCB) - Nifedipine Currently first line	Inhibit influx of calcium into cell and hence prevent myometrial contraction	20–30 mg, then 10–20 mg every 4–8 hours (max 90 mg/ day)	Maternal; Transient hypotension, headache and dizziness, Nausea Flushing Fetal/neonatal; None	Cardiac disease Hypotension Use with magnesium (collapse) Use with caution in renal disease
Atosiban - Oxytocin receptor antagonists Currently second line	Competitively inhibit oxytocin receptors	6.75 mg IV bolus, then 300 μg/ min every 3 hours. (max 45 hours)	Maternal; Minimal; Nausea and vomiting Hot flushes Hypotension and dizzness Fetal; None	None
Cyclo-oxygenase (COX) inhibitors Non-selective; indomethacin Selective (COX-2 inhibitor); sulindac nimesulide	Inhibition of COX leads to reduced PGs synthesis and hence myometrial relaxation	Indomethacin: 50–100 mg loading dose, then 25–50 mg every 6 hours for max 48 hours Sulindac: 200 mg every 12 hours for max 48 hours.	Maternal; Minimal if used for 48 hours; Less with COX2 inhibitors; Peptic ulcerations Thrombocytopenia Postpartum haemorrhage Allergic reaction. Fetal; Main concern; premature closure of ductus arteriosus Risk of neonatal necrotizing enterocolitis, IVH and renal dysfunction	Renal or hepatic disease Active peptic ulcer Uncontrolled hypertension NSAID-sensitive asthma and thrombocytopenia
Magnesium sulfate (MgSO4) Currently not in use	Intracellular calcium antagonist	Initial: 4–6 g/30 min, then: 2–4 g/h	Maternal; Headache and flushing Lethargy Muscle weakness and diplopia Dry mouth Pulmonary edema Fetal/neonatal; Lethargy Hypotonia Hypocalcemia Respiratory depression	Myasthenia gravis

Table 1.
Tocolytics.

8. B2-agonists

Ritodrine and other b-agonists as terbutaline, salbutamol were used as tocolytic agent but currently not recommeded as first line due to its maternal and neonatal side effects. They act on b2 receptors in myometrial smooth muscles via a cAMP dependent mechanism leading to reduction in the intracellular calcium causing muscular relaxation. Cochrane review on B2-agonists concluded that they decrease the number of preterm births within 48 hours but not within 7 days [1, 17, 18].

Maternal side effects include; palpitations and arrhythmias, chest pain, hypotension, flushing, nausea, headache, pulmonary oedema, hypokalaemia and hyperglycaemia. Neonatal side effects include; tachycardia, hypotension, hypoglycaemia, hypocalcemia and ileus. It is not proved that B2-agnosists are associated with neonatal periventericular haemorrhage [18].

9. Indomethacin

It is a nonsteroidal anti-inflamatory agent which inhibit cyclo-oxygenase enzyme and subsequently reduces myomeytrial prostaglandins concentration which inturn down regulates myometrial cells gap junctions, down regulates oxytocin receptors and reduces intracellular calcium levels. It has better tocolytic effect and better safety profile than b-agonists but its routine use is limited due to the associated fetal side effects [18].

Maternal side effects include; risks of peptic ulcerations, thrombocytopenia and postpartum haemorrhage and allergic reaction. Fetal side effects include; premature closure of ductus arteriosus. There is risk of neonatal necrotizing enterocolitis, intraventericular haemorrhage and renal dysfunction [18].

10. COX (cyclo-oxygenase)-2 inhibitors

It is a nonsteriodal anti-inflammatory agent which act specifically on cycloxgenase-2 enzyme which is upregulated in preterm labour. The mechanism of action is simillar to indomethacin but with better maternal side effect profile. Its routine use is limited due to fetal concerns over premature closure of the ductus and renal idysfunction [18].

11. Atosiban

Atosiban is an oxytocin analogue competitively blocks oxytocin and vasopressin receptors leading to reduced intracelluar calcium and lesser prostagladins production. It is recommended and licenced in preterm labour [1, 18, 19]. Its side effects include; maternal nausea, vomiting, hot flushes, hypotension and dizzness. It has simillar effectivness to B2-agonists and nifidipine but with a safer profile however, it is more expensive and given intravenously [1, 18].

12. Nifedipine

It is a calcium channel blocker that is proved to be effective in reducing preterm birth with lesser side effects compared to B2-agonists. It is admnistered orally and it is considered first line treatment option [1, 18]. The side effects of its use include; headache, dizzness, ankle odema, and constipation.

13. Magnesium sulphate

Cochrane review did not support its use for tocolysis as studies repeorted did not show that magnesium sulphate delayed or prevented preterm birth [18].

14. Antibiotics

The use of antibiotics is recommeded with preterm premature rupture of membranes (PPROM) based on ORACLE trial and chochrane review which proved that they reduce the time to delivery and the incidence of chorioamnionitis. They also decrease the ioccurance of neonatal sepsis and the need for neonatal surfactant and oxygen therapy. On the other hand; the ORACLE trial did not recommed its use in preterm labour without premature rupture of membranes as there was no difference in the neonatal outcomes [1, 20, 21].

It is also concluded that erythromycin is a better choice compared to coamoxiclav in women with preterm labour associated with premature rupture of membranes due to increased risk of necrotizing enetrocoilitis with the use of co-amoxiclav [20, 21].

15. Antenatal steriods

The Royal College of Obstetricians and Gynaecologists (RCOG) recommeded the use of antenatal corticosteriods in women with threating preterm labour as it is proven that their use has significant reduction in neonatal respiratory distress syndrome, intraventricular haemorrhage and neonatal death without increase in neonatal sepsis in women who has preterm labour and PPROM.

The use of antenatal steriods is recommeded with threatening preterm labour between 24 weeks and 34 weeks gestations may be considered up to 35 + 6 weeks with the optimal benefit within a window of one to seven days [1, 22].

The agent of choice is betamethasone as it has lesser risk of periventericular leucomalacia compared to the use of dexamethasone [22].

It is recommeded that betamethasone is adminstered intramuscularly in patients with preterm labour as the oral adminstration is associated with higher risk of neonatal sepsis and intraventricular haemorrhage. It is recommended to be used as two doses of 12 mg, 24 hours apart.

The use of mutiple courses of antenatal steriods is not recommeded as per RCOG guidance as it is associated with increassed risks of maternal osteoprosis, infection and imparied glucose tolerance. Multiple courses of steriods is associated with fetal risks including; intrauterine growth restriction, low birth weight, necrotizing enterocolitis, adrenal insufficiency and abnormal neurological development. Compared to a single course, mutiple courses have no benefit of improving neonatal respiratory distress syndrome, chronic lung disease and intraventericular haemorrhage [1, 22].

16. Magnisum sulphate for neuroprotection

Children born to women given magnesium sulphate for seizure prevention in severe pre-eclampsia were noted to have lower rates of cerebral palsy. This is possibly because magnisum decreases extracellular glutamate with hypoxia and hence reduces excitotoxicity. It also limits calcium influx through voltage-gated channels and in turn reduces the activation of apoptosis. Further more it reduces oxidative stress and reduces the production of pro-inflammatory cytokines.

It is use for neuroprotection is recommeded for use in women with established preterm labour or planned to hace elective preterm birth within 24 hours at gestations between 24 and 30 weeks. It is can be considered between 30 and 34 weeks [1, 23].

17. Mode of delivery

Vaginal delivery is considered to be appropriate choice in gestations under 24 weeks as the neonatal survival rate is very low. The challanging decision is the balance of vaginal delivery versus caesarean section in preterm delivery between 24 weeks and 37 weeks gestation [1, 24].

The decision for caesarean section is recommended to be for the obstetric reasons such as malpresentations and intrapartum fetal distress. Cochrane review for elective caesarean section in women with threating preterm labour between 24 and 37 weeks gestation has not shown statistically significant difference in the neonatal outcomes with regard the incidence of respiratory distress syndrome and neonatal seizures.

There is no evidence to support routine prophylactic outlet forceps or episiotomy when considering vaginal delivery between 24 and 37 weeks gestations. It is advisable to leave the fetal membranes intact till late in labour to reduce the risk of cord prolapse. The fetal scalp electrode and fetal blood sampling use is contraindicated prior to 34 weeks gestation and hence any suspicious fetal monitoring trace should be considered as indication for caesarean section. Their use is considered between 34 and 36 weeks gestation. It is also important to note that ventouse delivery is contraindicated prior to 34 weeks gestation. Consideration should be taken for caesarean section in preterm delivery with breech presentation [1, 24].

Delayed cord clamping for at least 30 seconds but no longer than three minutes is advisable in preterm deliveries to allow auto transfusion of the baby. Senior obstetrician should be consulted in planning the delivery and the decision-making throughout the labour [1, 24].

Parents should have discussion with joint obstetric and neonatal team prior embarking onto labour is helpful to ensure their understanding of challenges for the preterm baby such as ability to maintain stable core body temperature, ability to breath spontaneously and feeding difficulties. The expected postnatal care for the preterm baby should be planned as detailed as possible with the parents and ensure the availability of the facilities.

Author details

Maged Shendy[1]*, Hend Hendawy[2], Amr Salem[2], Ibrahim Alatwi[3] and Abdurahman Alatawi[3]

1 King Khaled Hospital, Tabuk, Kingdom of Saudi Arabia

2 Basildon Hospital, United Kingdom

3 Pharmaceutical Care Adminsteration, Tabuk Region, Kingdom of Saudi Arabia

*Address all correspondence to: mego_marmar@yahoo.com

References

[1] NICE guideline Preterm labour and birth [NG25] Published date: 20 November 2015 Last updated: 02 August 2019

[2] Brocklehurst P, Gordon A, Heatley E, Milan SJ. Antibiotics for treating bacterial vaginosis in pregnancy. Cochrane Database Syst Rev 2013; (1): CD000262.

[3] Sangkomkamhang US, Lumbiganon P, Prasertcharoensuk W, Laopaiboon M. Antenatal lower genital tract infection screening and treatment programs for preventing preterm delivery.Cochrane Database Syst Rev 2015; (5): CD006178.

[4] Royal College of Obstetricians and Gynaecologists. Cervical Cerclage. Green-top Guideline No. 60. London: RCOG, 2011.

[5] Sotiriadis A, Papatheodorou S, KavvadiasA,MakrydimasG.Transvaginal cervical length measurement for prediction of preterm birth in women with threatened preterm labor: a meta-analysis. Ultrasound Obstet Gynecol 2010; 35: 54-64.

[6] Alfirevic Z, Stampalija T, Roberts D, Jorgensen AL. Cervical stitch (cerclage) for preventing preterm birth in singleton pregnancy. Cochrane Database Syst Rev 2012; (4): CD008991.

[7] Deshpande SN, van Asselt AD, Tomini F, et al. Rapid fetal fibronectin testing to predict preterm birth in women with symptoms of premature labour: a systematic review and cost analysis. Health Technol Assess 2013; 17: 1-138.

[8] Menon R, Torloni MR, Voltolini C, et al. Biomarkers of spontaneous preterm birth: an overview of the literature in the last four decades. Reprod Sci 2011; 18: 1046-70.

[9] Moore T, Hennessy EM, Myles J, et al. Neurological and developmental outcome in extremely preterm children born in England in 1995 and 2006: the EPICure studies. BMJ 2012; 345: e7961.

[10] Royal College of Obstetricians and Gynaecologists. Perinatal Management of Pregnant Women at the Threshold of Infant Viability: the Obstetric Perspective. Scientific Impact Paper No. 41. London: RCOG, 2014.

[11] Berghella V, Rafael TJ, Szychowski JM, Rust OA, Owen J. Cerclage for short cervix on ultrasonography in women with singleton gestations and previous preterm birth: a metaanalysis.Obstet Gynecol 2011; 117: 663-71.

[12] Di Renzo GC, Roura LC, Facchinetti F, et al. Guidelines for the management of spontaneous preterm labor: identification of spontaneous preterm labor, diagnosis of preterm premature rupture of membranes, and preventive tools for preterm birth. J Matern Fetal Neonatal Med 2011; 24: 659-67.

[13] Royal College of Obstetricians and Gynaecologists. The Use of Progesterone to Prevent Preterm Delivery. 2015.

[14] Dodd J, Jones L, Flenady V, Cincotta R, Crowther C. Prenatal administration of progesterone for preventing preterm birth in women considered to be at risk of preterm birth. Cochrane. Database Syst Rev 2013; (7): CD004947.

[15] Goya M, Pratcorona L, Merced C, et al.; Pesario Cervical para Evitar Prematuridad (PECEP) Trial Group. Cervical pessary in pregnant women with a short cervix (PECEP): an open-label randomised controlled trial. Lancet 2012; 379: 1800-6.

[16] Sosa CG, Althabe F, Belizan JM, Bergel E. Bed rest in singleton pregnancies for preventing preterm birth. Cochrane Database Syst Rev 2015; (3): CD003581.

[17] Flenady V, Wojcieszek AM, Papatsonis DN, et al. Calcium channel blockers for inhibiting preterm labour and birth. Cochrane Database Syst Rev 2014; (6): CD002255.

[18] Royal College of Obstetricians and Gynaecologists. Tocolysis for Women in Preterm Labour. Green-top Guideline No. 1b. London: RCOG, February 2011.

[19] Flenady V, Reinebrant HE, Liley HG, Tambimuttu EG, Papatsonis DN. Oxytocin receptor antagonists for inhibiting preterm labour. Cochrane Database Syst Rev 2014; (6): CD004452.

[20] Kenyon SL, Taylor DJ, Tarnow-Mordi W; ORACLE Collaborative Group. Broad-spectrum antibiotics for preterm, prelabour rupture of fetal membranes: the ORACLE I randomized trial. Lancet 2001; 357: 979-88.

[21] Royal College of Obstetricians and Gynaecologists. Preterm Prelabour Rupture of Membranes. Green-top Guideline No. 44. London: RCOG, October 2010.

[22] Royal College of Obstetricians and Gynaecologists. Antenatal Corticosteroids to Reduce Neonatal Morbidity. Green-top Guideline No. 7. London: RCOG, October 2010.

[23] Royal College of Obstetricians and Gynaecologists. Magnesium Sulphate to Prevent Cerebral Palsy Following Preterm Birth. Scientific Impact Paper No. 29. London: RCOG, 2011.

[24] Alfirevic Z, Milan SJ, Livio S. Caesarean section versus vaginal delivery for preterm birth in singletons. Cochrane Database Syst Rev 2013; (9): CD000078.

Chapter 4

Identification and Management of High Risk Complications during Postnatal Period by Ground Level Workers

Jasneet Kaur and Suresh Ray

Abstract

What to expect after the child birth. A healthy newborn is considered as priority, but postnatal care counts too. It is not always that story ended up with safe child birth; mother is still at high risk if not taken care after birth. Antenatal and intra natal period are the hardest part of a life span of a pregnant women. Mandatory Antenatal visits and maternal and child health services provided by the government with hand holding national programs and schemes have converted this tough path into smooth platform. Similarly postnatal period is equally important in the life of a new mother. The transition has already been set up by creating fourth stage of pregnancy instead of traditional three stages. Several studies have observed complications in postnatal period especially Primary PPH but very minimal studies had concentrated on Secondary PPH. Over and above there are no significant and standardized guidelines made available for the health workers to define the set limits of blood loss and management of secondary PPH. The condition becomes more critical when severe secondary PPH came for the hospitalization when the exact cause and associated factors remains often unknown. Also many postpartum infections emerge 24 hours after the delivery and discharge from hospital. Consequently, in the lack of proper knowledge and skills regarding identification of postnatal complications like secondary PPH and Puerperal infection, many cases go undiagnosed and unreported. This chapter will deals with the skills of the ground level workers required to identify and manage selected high risk complications in postnatal period.

Keywords: PPH, Puerperal Infections, Knowledge, Skills, Ground level workers

1. Introduction

High Risk mothers in the postnatal period are those mothers who are at the risk of their lives because of the complication occurs in the postnatal periods. These complications are usually life threatening if not treated at the earliest [1].

Antenatal and intra natal period are the hardest part of a life span of a pregnant women. Mandatory Antenatal visits and Maternal and Child Health services provided by the government with hand holding national programs and schemes have converted this tough path into safe and smooth platform [1].

Similarly postnatal period is equally important in the life of a new mother. The transition has already been set up by creating fourth stage of pregnancy instead of traditional three stages.

It's not always over subsequent to delivery. Still a successful delivery can put the mother into High risk Situations. Mother has to face many challenges in Postnatal Period. The major cause of Maternal Mortality Rate are the Postnatal conditions of which lays the mothers into high risk conditions like Postpartum Haemorrhage, Postpartum Eclampsia, Puerperal Infections etc. Major Maternal health challenges in the postpartum period [2]. There are many factors associated with that especially the cases which are unidentified. The lack of knowledge as well as skill to identify and mange is the prime concern. As soon as mother discharge from the hospital after two days one should not presume that things are over. Therefore Post-natal visits are planned by the government to follow up the mothers as they are still at the risk of getting complications which can be life threatening [2].

The postnatal period is defined as the first six weeks after birth and is considered as one of the critical periods for the health as well as survival of the mother and her neonate. It is the most critical time for both mother and child during labour and moments after delivery up till puerperium. Negligence in detecting crucial symptoms and care during this period can result into death and disability [2].

The World Health Organization (WHO) described that the postnatal period is one of the most dangerous and still most neglected period during the life of the mother. Maximum number of the maternal and neonatal deaths happens to be in this period especially in first 24 hours [1] and 66% occur during the first week [3].

Reports of maternal mortality across the globe indicate the maximum number of deaths of women is from complications which are al the most supplementary to postnatal problems, and not merely antenatal problems and problems ascending throughout the birthing process [3]. That is why Government is making mandatory protocol of postnatal visits. A complete assessment is in post-partum period suggested in 12 weeks for assurance. The suggestive care should primarily emphasis on immediate requirements and high risks for morbidity and mortality. After that the process of care should be shifted for chronic conditions, maintenance and rehabilitation. Initial Postnatal visits should assess problems from pregnancy as well as common high risk postpartum complications. Following care should focus a full bio psychosocial assessment and other needs for further problems [3].

These indicators are more than enough to suggest the importance and significance of postnatal time period.

A Substantial growth strategy has been tried and implemented globally to improve maternal health. 72% of women delivered with the help of skilled personnel around the world, and the maternal mortality ratio also has decreased considerably 210 per 1 lakh live births. The condition is not same across. South East Asia and in the sub Saharan part of Africa only 67% of women go for skilled assistance deliveries [3]. Postnatal care has reached across the world but hardly a smaller amount women usually receive standard postnatal care visit within 2 days after postpartum period [4]. The same has been justified by the investigation of Demographic and Health Survey data which was obtained from 23 sub-Saharan African countries which stated that barely 13 percent of the women had received care within 2 days of postnatal period [4].

The guidelines on postnatal care released globally for mothers and new-borns has recently been updated by World Health Organisation through a technical consultation process. These guidelines addressed and emphasised upon the time and activities to be done for the postnatal care for mothers and new-borns and focused on settings which has limited resources especially in the in low and the middle income group of countries [4]. They emphasised the additional references which are meant for on maternal, perinatal and new-born health [5]. They also elaborated the recommendations which are exclusively meant for type of health care worker who can practice safety measures for delivery and new-born health care interventions [6].

It is not always over after delivery. Even a successful delivery can put the mother into High risk Situations. Mother may have to face many challenges in Postnatal Period. The major cause of Maternal Mortality Rate are the Postnatal conditions of which lays the mothers into high risk conditions like Postpartum Haemorrhage, Postpartum Eclampsia, Puerperal Infections etc. are health challenges in the postpartum period.

2. High risk postpartum complications

Postpartum period is usually bifurcated in three phases; the initial or acute phase, which is the period between 6 to 12 hours after delivery; sub acute phase, which lasts for about 2 to 6 weeks after delivery, and the delayed phase, which can last up to six months [19]. Near about 87–94% of women report at least one major health issue in sub-acute phase [20]. Almost 31% of women reported problems in late Phase [7].

2.1 Acute phase

The common complications in the acute phase are Post partum hemorrhage, Perineal pain. Post partum hemorrhage is one of the high risk complication.

Postpartum haemorrhage is a condition which involves loss of blood which usually takes place within the 24 hours after the childbirth. The hours are considered to be the most critical in assessing the abnormal bleeding [7].

2.2 Subacute phase

The common complication Puerperal genital infection, Post partum Eclamsia, HELLP syndrome, Post partum urinary incontinence, Fouls smelling lochia, Post partum depression and stress. In this phase the infection may leads to sepsis also.

Puperal genital infection is one of the post-natal complication in displayed with symptoms of fever accompanied by chills and foul smelling vaginal discharge. It involves an inclusive range of postpartum infections which are caused by bacteria and involves interior of the uterus or the genital tract as common sites. There are few other also like Post-natal depression, Breast engorgement etc. Out of these Postpartum Haemorrhage and Puerperal Infection are leading the board.

Postpartum Eclampsia is a condition where mother have high blood pressure and Proteinuria along with the additional symptoms which includes headache, pain in the upper abdomen and visual disturbances [8].

2.3 Delayed phase

The complications in delayed phase are Fecal incontinence, Pelvic Prolapse Post partum thyroiditis etc.

Postpartum Haemorrhage (PPH) is the extreme abnormal bleeding which happens after the childbirth. Bleeding within the limits is normal after the childbirth but the major worry and distress arises when the loss of blood is more than 500 ml after normal vaginal delivery and 1000 ml in caesarean after the expulsion of the placenta [7].

Primary Post-Partum Haemorrhage is when the bleeding happens to be within first 24 hours after the delivery whereas any excessive and abnormal bleeding which happens after 24 hours and up till 6 weeks after the delivery is called secondary Post-Partum Haemorrhage [9].

Across the globe about 1.2 per cent of the deliveries are some or other way correlated to the Post-Partum Haemorrhage especially in the developing countries. Out of those almost 3% of the women die because of this cause. This complication has taken the score board to 30% deaths of women in India [10].

Post-Partum haemorrhage (PPH) occurs quite frequently after delivery. The incidence of PPH after the vaginal delivery has been reported between 2 to 4 and same after caesarean section accounts to 6 percent [8]. OverallPost-Partum haemorrhage accounts 28% for the maternal mortality in developing countries and 13% maternal deaths in high income countries and if counted worldwide it is 35% [10].

Secondary postpartum haemorrhage is classically defined as haemorrhage in excess of lochia occurring after the 24 hours of the delivery up till six weeks of the post-partum. The rationale behind differentiating these two types of PPH lies in the fact that the predominant causes leading to these are different. Uterine atony is the most common cause of primary postpartum haemorrhage, retained products of conception cause secondary PPH most of the time [10].

Secondary postpartum haemorrhage (PPH) is a condition wherein excessive abnormal vaginal bleeding happens after twenty four hours of the delivery up to 6 weeks of the postpartum period. Primary postpartum haemorrhage has clear cut defining limits of the blood loss whereas on the other side, Secondary PPH doesn't have a clear idea and standard defined limits for quantity of the blood loss. The clinical language of Secondary PPH varies from increased lochia to immense bleeding. Therefore diagnosis is sometimes subjective in nature which leads to frequent variations in recorded incidence. Some times for the mothers also it is very difficult to decide whether they are having secondary PPH or not [11].

Secondary PPH can be caused by numerous other etiological factors, the significant among which are, primary sub involution of placental bed, endometritis, pseudoanuerysm of the uterine artery, non-union of uterine incision etc. [10–13] Other rare causes of PPH have also been reported [12, 13]. There is ample data exists in the available literature exploring the primary PPH but secondary PPH has not been considered and explored with similar enthusiasm. The reason is simply because secondary PPH is not perceived to contribute much to the maternal mortality and morbidity. Data from Indian subcontinent is sparse [14].

Another one of the important postnatal complication which put the mother into high risk is Puerperal Infection. A puerperal infection happens when bacteria contaminate the uterus and its surrounding areas after a woman gives birth.

Puerperal Infection is counted as the third most critical reason for the deaths of the mothers of across worldwide after haemorrhage and abortion. World Health Organization (WHO) has estimated that this complication accounts for 15% of the all maternal deaths annually. It is the 6th leading cause of the global burden of the diseases in women in reproductive age groups especially in low and middle income countries. This complication leads to enduring health problems in later life of women like pelvic inflammatory disease, and infertility. It usually happens as infection of the genital tract during postpartum period along with the symptoms of Fever more than 101°F, pain in the pelvic region, foul smelling vaginal discharge may or may not include pus, and slow or delayed involution of the uterus. It is a more generic than puerperal sepsis as it comprises all extra-genital infections and other incidental infections along with puerperal sepsis [15].

Sample Registration System in India estimated that almost 11% maternal deaths happened in the year 2011–2013 were due to puerperal sepsis [16]. As per population based study in rural areas of Maharashtra state puerperal sepsis was leading on the second number as major cause of maternal mortality with the figures of 13.2% followed by postpartum haemorrhage and same has been found 12% in Pune [16].

Puerperal infection is very much preventable. An effective provision of sufficient antenatal care, a quick and effective referral system and on dot time availability of the early management and treatment are mandate for the prevention.

Similarly a very rarest complication can emerged called Postpartum Eclampsia. This is the condition which usually emerged with 48 hours of post-partum period and sometimes after 48 hours which is often called late onset of Postpartum Eclampsia [8]. The warning sign includes stomach pain, headache, vision changes and shortness of breath. It's significant to identify that delivery is not the end point for preeclampsia rather woman can develop preeclampsia the delivery also, despite the status of high blood pressure during her pregnancy [8].

The immense role of community health workers in the health care system is considered as one of the crucial component to comply with the targeted goals of the health care sector.

Nursing training in India starts with the certificate and diploma courses and went up to graduate, Postgraduate and Doctorate levels. The most common levels found in the first Health Visitors.

3. Role of ground level health workers

The Rural sector in India is mostly taken care by First level of Health care delivery system which are Sub centres, Primary Health centres and Rural Health Centres. The major Nursing health task force working in the field are Auxiliary Nurse Midwives (ANMs) and Local Health Visitors (LHVs). These are mostly responsible for the postnatal visits at home and will do the follow up. They assess the mothers and deliver need base care [17].

Post-natal care has transformed unexpectedly over the past many years. The time period in the Maternity areas has been reduced progressively from one week to two days. After that either the mother has to come up to the health centres for the follow up or the Ground level health task force i.e. ANMs or LHVs has to extend the doorstep health service for them those who aren't/can't come to the centre [18].

The ANMs and LHVs are the first baseline and front workers who develops the bond and interact with the mother when she go back home after the delivery, even after the one week of the childbirth [19]. This period is a very much susceptible time to relook the things with new challenges with baby. Women need someone with whom she can contact for required information and adequate support. The body, mind and social changes may signify certain hurdles and challenges for the women concerned after the delivery. Lack of proper knowledge, information and support may be very dangerous as it may lead to endanger mother's life. The abnormal sign and symptoms may appear normal to the mother and she may not able to identify those as serious complications. This lead to increase the risk of morbidly and mortality [19].

Immediate complications after the delivery are usually taken care by the Hospital/Health centre staff as mother stays at the health care facilities up till 48 hours. Many times mothers don't come for the Postnatal Follow up at the health centre. At this point of time ANMs and LHVs do visit their homes and do the assessment.

The ground level nursing cadre plays an imperative part in the identification and management of complications arises when mothers leave hospital and goes to their homes but they are still in the postnatal period. Therefore the complete onus lies on their shoulders to bring the high risk mothers into the picture [20].

Though government has taken the initiatives and Skill birth attendant programs but still gaps are available. Many studies had been piloted to recognize the level of knowledge and skills in the past for health care workers especially ANMs LHVs, and even skill birth attendants. According to study conducted by WHO [15] stating the level and knowledge of skilled workers in maternity areas and extended the ways forwards too. The study results explained that professional nurses have 57% and auxiliary nurses have 51% knowledge asked as per the knowledge questionnaire. As far as skill is concerned the scores for these groups falls at the level of 64% and results were statistically significant at 0.001. The way forward recommended by WHO is to bridge the identified gaps in competency levels and enhance the training levels for better results [15].

4. Knowledge and skills of ground level workers regarding identification and management of high risk complications

In case of India, every five women die every hour, and nearly 45,000 mothers die due to causes related to Postpartum and Postnatal period every year in India which accounts for 17 per cent of such deaths globally" [21].

National Family Health Survey-4, recommended the strategy for the quality facility and service that is confirming the mandatory postnatal care to be imparted within first twenty four hours of delivery followed by the on 3rd, 7th, 14th and 42nd day home visit subsequently to identify and manage the emergent complications which occurs in the occurring postnatal period. Therefore Auxiliary nurse mid-wives, Lady Health Visitors, and other cadre of nurses working in the first referral units and PHCs are meant to be focused on and proficient for handling these conditions in the respective home visits [22].

Women's death with Post-Partum Haemorrhage is an important indicator for the maternal health which helps anyone to reflect upon the kind of care been imparted to the mothers during the intrapartum and postpartum period. Many of this kind of negligence are preventable. In many situations, deaths due to high rates of post-partum haemorrhage complications are associated with the gap in the health care system, along with the factors like inadequate information and skills of health care workers in the prevention of PPH and its quick management, lack of decision making ability of health workers at appropriate time and which leads to delays in further referral system [23].

Another problem is that be that many postpartum infections emerges 24 after the delivery and the discharge from the hospital. Consequently, in the lack proper knowledge and skills regarding identification of postnatal complications like secondary PPH and Puerperal Infection during postnatal follow-up, many cases of identification of High risk mothers can go undiagnosed and unreported. This will add on to the burden of increased maternal Mortality rate, where on the other side these can be easily detectable and managed if appropriate knowledge and skills are used.

A study conducted at in North-East district of Delhi among 55 ASHA workers on their Knowledge and practice for maternal healthcare delivery in Delhi. The results showed that ASHAs workers possess substantially good knowledge but the practices are not up to the level. The reason identified as various problems challenged by them which require immediate addressing by skill based trainings including decent communication and ability to solve the problems. Over and above vigilant supervision should be considered a primary fragment of work practice during the practice to safeguard that imparted knowledge is appropriately giving the required results in the form of good practices [24].

The identification and initial management of High risk mother during the post-natal period is totally depends upon the knowledge and skills of these ground level workers, otherwise they will remain un-notified and unreported. The question arise is how far the health task force is skilled and possess accurate information. Government is nowhere less than any other by providing extreme measures and resources to train them. Still the gaps in the knowledge and skills are there. It also depends on the mode of learning and training they got which is one of the biggest reasons for inadequate training. The hands on live demonstration training sessions in these cases are highly recommended.

5. Mandatory skills to be performed by ground level workers

5.1 Post natal visits and examination

There should be minimum 4 Postnatal Visits as follows. **Table 1** depicts the crux of the postnatal visits.

5.1.1 First visit: 1st day (within 24 hours)

The first 48 hours are the most crucial hours in the whole life span of Post partum period. Major Post partum complications like PPH and eclampsia, occur during this period. These complications cannot be ignored as considered to be the most fatal one and are leading causes of maternal mortality rate [25].

Therefore a mother who just delivered must be closely watched uptill at least 48 hours. It is the duty of ground level workers to inform the woman about the criticality of the complications, and rationale for the stay in the health care facility for at least 48 hours. During this time period required care should be provided to her. Ground level worker must put emphasis on that this is very much important for her well being and baby too [25].

If the delivery is conducted at Sub center/at home, ANM should visit to the newly delivered mother with in the first 24 hours of the delivery [25].

She should ask the mother for the discharge or delivery card. This card contains the data and information pertaining to the antenatal visits and delivery details [26].

- After this first she should ask her history.
- Do physical assessment and examination.
- If the delivery has been conducted at home, then ask the details from the support services at the time of delivery or the person present during the delivery.

Visits	After Delivery at Sub Centre	After Delivery at Primary health centre/First Referral Unit
1st Visit	1st Day (within 24 Hours)	Not Required as women discharged after 48 hours*
2nd Visit	3rd day after delivery	3rd day after delivery
3rd Visit	7th day after delivery	7th day after delivery
4th Visit	6 weeks after delivery	6 weeks after delivery

**Why First 48 Hours are important after delivery?*

Table 1.
Details of the Postnatal Visits.

- If the delivery is not conducted by the skilled birth attendant, but a person of close relative or the one who accompanied her during the postpartum period, then inform her reading the complications in future which may arise.
- She should explain about all signs and symptoms so that earlier can be informed to the health care facility and relevant actions can be taken earliest to prevent the further complications [25].

Things to do at First Visit:

1. History Taking: Ask the mother
    - The place and location of the delivery.
    - The individual who conducted the delivery?
    - Ask about any complications happens during the delivery,
    - Any bleeding Per vagina
    - The number of pads soaked with blood),
    - Any convulsions or loss of consciousness
    - Leg pain or abdominal pain
    - Fever
    - Retention of urine or dribbling,
    - Any breast tenderness, etc. [27]

Other than that ask the mother

- Whether breast feeding has been started?
- Whether mother has resumed her normal or regular diet?

Examination

Assess the following

- Assess the pulse, blood pressure, temperature and respiratory rate.
- Pallor skin.
- Abdominal examination for the uterus assessment. Usually, the uterus will be contracted, round and hard.
- If the uterus is soft that states its tenderness and in this case refer her to the First Referral Unit.
- Look for any tear in Vulva and perineum

DOI: http://dx.doi.org/10.5772/intechopen.97533

- Swelling or discharge or Pus.
- Check the count of pads for assessment of blood loss.
- Check the color and smell of Lochia. If it is foul smelling, it can be the signs of puerperal sepsis. If this be the case then, refer the woman to the First Referral Unit.
- Check the breasts for any tenderness or presence of lumps,
- Assess the nipples and pattern of breastfeeding. If the woman has any complaint regarding this, refer her to the First Referral Unit [27].

Counselling:

Hygiene

- Washing of Perineum
- Changing Pads every 4 – 6hrly
- Hand Washing before handling the baby
- Bathe Daily
- Rooming In with baby

Nutrition

- Good intake of fluid and food intake
- Nutritious diet with more calories
- Avoid Heavy work

Contraception

- Birth Spacing methods
- Avoid sexual contact till 6 week of puerperium

Breast feeding

- Breast feeding within one hour of birth
- Feed Colostrum
- Exclusive breast feeding
- Feed on both breast
- Warm compress on Breast if engorged.

IFA supplement

- If Hb level is <11 g/dl, then mother should take two Iron and Folic Acid tablets once in a day for 3 months.
- After 1 month if the Hemoglobin level doesn't increase refer her to Primary Health Centre
- If Hemoglobin level is less than 7 g/dl refer to First Referral Unit [27].

5.1.2 Second and third post natal visit: 3rd day after delivery and 7th day after delivery

Assessment and examination

- Assess the Temperature, pulse, and blood pressure.
- Assess for the pallor.
- Assess the uterus, for the contracted wall. If it is not hard and round then refer the women to First Referral Unit.
- Assess any kind of tear at vulva and perineum. Check the swelling and pus at the site.If yes, then refer the mother to First Referral Unit.
- Check the pad for bleeding.
- Examine the colour and smell of Lochia. If it is more and foul smelling then refer her to the First Referral Unit.
- Breast examination should be done for any lump or tenderness. it that be the case, it may be the sign of Infection, then refer the mother to First Referral Unit [26].

Care
Diet and rest

- Ground level workers should check for the diet of the mother during postnatal period. Mother should be advised to take the diet which is rich in calories, iron, proteins, and vitamins as required by the lactating mother. Micro-nutrients and milk products should be added.
- Green vegetables, pulses, meat, eggs, fish and poultry must be added in the diet.
- Groundnuts, and *ragi,* jiggery need to considered in the plate as rich in iron.
- Fruits need to added to add on fiber in the diet [26].

Contraception

- Family planning is the important component in Postnatal period. Ground level workers while visit at home should ask mother about her resuming the periods, so that contraception can be planned.

- Mother should be explained with the various methods of family planning available [27].

5.1.3 Fourth post natal visit: 6 weeks after delivery

Assessment and examination

- Vaginal bleeding should be stopped by this time.
- Assess the vital signs especially blood pressure.
- Check for the sign of pallor.
- Assess for vulva or perineal tear
- Assess for any swelling or signs of pus.
- Breast examination for tenderness or lumps.
- If presence of above signs, refer her to the Primary health centre/First Referral unit [27].

Care

Emphasize the importance of using contraceptive methods for spacing or limiting the size of the family [27].

6. Management of high risk areas by ground level workers

6.1 Retained placenta and placental fragments

The placenta is said to be retained if it is not delivered within half an hour of the birth ofthe baby. Bleeding may or may not occur in cases of retained placenta.

Retained placental fragments or pieces of membrane will cause PPH. This can be suspected if a portion of the maternal surface of the placenta is missing or the membranes with their vessels are torn. If placenta is partially separated or retained then it will cause continuous vaginal bleeding which further leads to PPH. Manage such cases as in the case of PPH [27].

- If the placenta is already separated and is lying at the tip of the birth canal, then gently remove it.
- If it is not separated, then DONOT ATTEMPT THIS PROCEDURE. Refer the mother to First Referral Unit [27].

6.2 Puerperal sepsis

It is the infection of the genital tract from the time rupture of membranes or labor and till 42 days after delivery. Any two or more of the following signs and symptoms are present.

- Presence of Fever >38°C

- Abdominal pain at the lower end aln with tenderness
- Foul-smelling lochia
- Burning urination
- Uterus not contracted
- Weakness
- Continuous Vaginal bleeding

Fever in the Postnatal period can occur because of the causes other than puerperal sepsis like mastitis, non obstetric causes or may be Urinary tract infection (UTI) etc. [27]

In this case, combination of antibiotics is given for at least 48 hours with following regime.

- Inj. Ampicillin 2 g IV every 6 hours,
- Inj Gentamicin 5 mg/kg body weight (IV) every 24 hours,
- Metronidazole 500 mg IV every 8 hours.
- If fever still persists 72 hours after starting the antibiotic then refer to the Medical officer for further treatment [28].

Oral antibiotics are not necessary after stopping IV antibiotics.

6.3 Vaginal and perineal tears

There are four degrees of tears:

- First-degree tear: This type of tear happens in the vaginal mucosa and connective tissues.
- Second-degree tear: This tear involves the vaginal mucosa, connective tissues and underlying muscles.
- Third-degree tear: It involves complete coverage of the anal sphincter.
- Fourth degree tear: This tear encroaches the rectal mucosa [26].

Ground level workers must distinguish the superficial (first-degree) and deep tears [26].

6.4 They are only permitted to manage first-degree tears

- Superficial tear which is not bleeding requires no suturing. As a measure the area needs to be cleaned and cover with a clean pad.
- Superficial tear which is bleeding, requires pressure on the site for some time, at least for 10–15 minutes. It will control the bleeding.

- Deep perineal tears (2nd, 3rd and 4th degree): Refer the mother to a 24 hour First Referral Unit.

- Before referring the mother, cover the tear with a sterile pad or gauze. Positioned the legs together. Do not cross the ankles.

- In case of heavy bleeding and degree of tear can be diagnosed and decide upon, put a pad into the vaginal cavity and refer the woman to the First Referral Unit.

- Immediately establish an IV line and infuse fluids rapidly. To prevent the Shock, raise the foot end. Keep the woman warm during transportation [26].

6.5 Post Partum Hemorrhage (PPH)

The ground level worker should react immediately once it has been realized that the amount of blood flow is exceeding the limits, She should immediately do the following.

Figure 1 depict the protocols to be followed by the ground level health workers in management of Primary and secondary PPH.

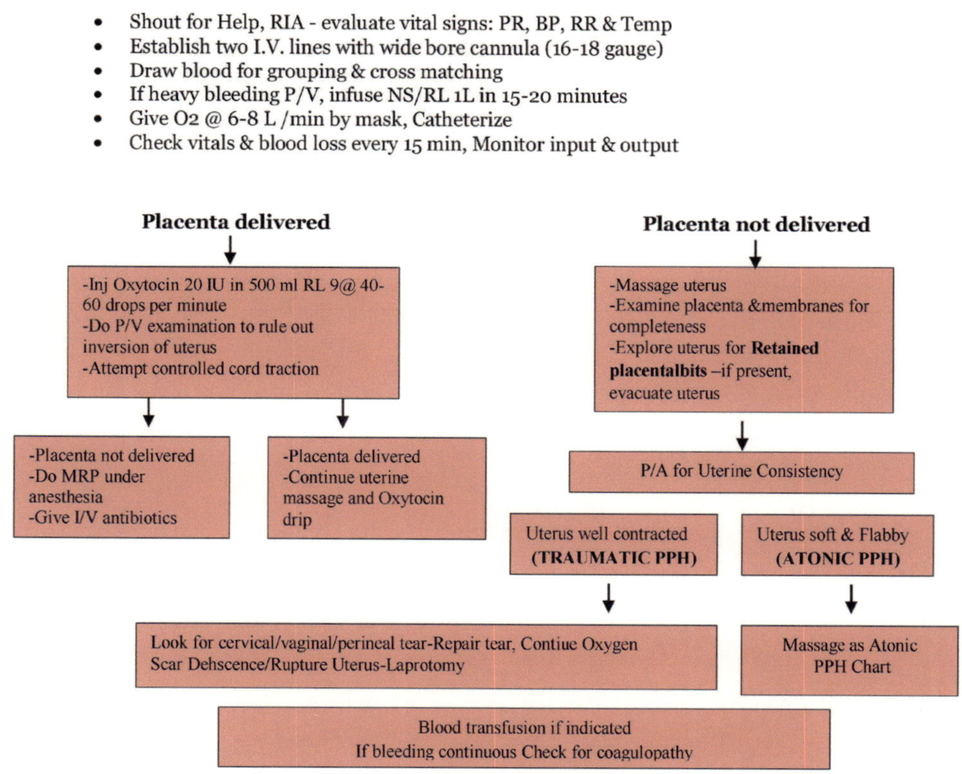

Figure 1.
Protocol to be followed for management of PPH.

7. Conclusion

This chapter concludes that the health task force though assumed to be well trained as per the qualification mandates still requires an updates and practice on hands on skill trainings rather than the traditional lecture cum discussion methods. Health task force must be abreast with the knowledge and skills. Though Government is taking every effort to train the workers and hand hold them but there is a strong need to modify the strategies and implementation process where the skill enhancement should be given a huge importance especially in the complicated situation where the onus totally lies on the ground level workers to identify and manage the complications before getting critical. The training received by the ground level workers needs to be streamlined and the skills needs to be enhanced time to time with updated practices. The strategic reforms are quite necessary to shed off the traditional classroom lectures.

Author details

Jasneet Kaur[1]* and Suresh Ray[2]

1 Symbiosis College of Nursing, Symbiosis International (Deemed University), Pune, India

2 Bharati Vidyapeeth College of Nursing, Bharati Vidyapeeth (Deemed to Be University), Pune, India

*Address all correspondence to: jasneetkaur@scon.edu.in

References

[1] Every New-born, An Executive Summary for The Lancet's Series. May 2014.

[2] Nour NM. An introduction to maternal mortality. Rev Obstetrics and Gynaecology. 2008 spring; 1(2):77-81. PMID: 18769668; PMCID: PMC2505173

[3] WHO. 2014. World Health Statistics 2014. Geneva: WHO

[4] Warren C, Daly P, Toure L, and Mongi P. Postnatal Care. Opportunities for Africa's New-borns: Practical Data Policy and Programmatic Support for New-born Care in Africa. 2006; 79-90

[5] WHO. 2013. Recommendations on Maternal and Perinatal Health. Geneva: WHO. Guidelines on maternal, new-born, child and adolescent health approved by the WHO guidelines review committee.

[6] WHO recommends optimizing health worker roles to improve access to key maternal and new-born health interventions through task shifting; WHO, 2012.

[7] Borders N. After the afterbirth: a critical review of postpartum health relative to method of delivery. Journal of Midwifery & Women's Health. 2006; 51 (4): 242-248

[8] Minnerup J, Kleffner I, Wersching H, Zimmermann J, Schäbitz WR, Niederstadt T, Dziewas R. Late Onset Postpartum Eclampsia: It is Really Never Too Late-A Case of Eclampsia 8 Weeks after Delivery. Stroke Res Treat. 2010; 2010:798616. doi: 10.4061/2010/798616. Epub 2009 Sep 1. PMID: 20798839; PMCID: PMC2925215

[9] Amy JJ. Severe Postpartum Haemorrhage: A Rational Approach. National Medical Journal Indian. 1998; 11:86-8.

[10] Khan KS. WHO Analysis of Causes of Maternal Death: A Systematic Review. The Lancet. 2006; 367:1066-74.

[11] Dossou M, Debost-Legrand A, Déchelotte P LémeryD, Vendittelli F. Severe secondary postpartum haemorrhage: a historical cohort. Birth. 2015; 42(2):149-55.

[12] Nanda S, Singhal S, Sharma D, Sood M, Singhal SK. Nonunion of uterine incision: a rare cause of secondary postpartum haemorrhage: a report of 2 cases. AustN Z J Obstet-Gynaecol. 1997; 37(4):475-6.

[13] Larsen JV,Janowski K, Krolilowski A Secondary post-partum haemorrhage due to uterine wound dehiscence. Cent African Journal of Med. 1995;41(9):294-6

[14] Kelly SM, Belli AM, Campbell S. Hoveyda F. Arteriovenous malformation of the uterus associated with secondary postpartum haemorrhage. Ultrasound Obstet. Gynecol. 2003;21(6):602-5

[15] www.who.int/healthinfo/statistics/bod_maternalsepsis.pdf. 2020.

[16] planningcommission.nic.in/aboutus/committee/strgrp/stgp_fmlywel/sgfw. 2020

[17] Pyone T, Karvande S, Gopalakrishnan S, Purohit V, Nelson S, Balakrishnan SS, Mistry N, Mathai M. Factors governing the performance of Auxiliary Nurse Midwives in India: A study in Pune district. PLoS One. 2019 Dec 27; 14(12):e0226831. doi: 10.1371/journal.pone.0226831. PMID: 31881071; PMCID: PMC6934276.

[18] Counselling for Maternal and Newborn Health Care: A Handbook for Building Skills. Geneva: World Health Organization; 2013. 11, POSTNATAL CARE OF THE MOTHER AND NEWBORN. Available from: https://

www.ncbi.nlm.nih.gov/books/NBK304191/

[19] Finlayson K, Crossland N, Bonet M, Downe S. What matters to women in the postnatal period: A meta-synthesis of qualitative studies. PLoS One. 2020 Apr 22; 15(4):e0231415. doi: 10.1371/journal.pone.0231415. PMID: 32320424; PMCID: PMC7176084.

[20] Jauniaux E, Chantraine F, Silver RM, Langhoff-Roos J; FIGO Placenta Accreta Diagnosis and Management Expert Consensus Panel. FIGO consensus guidelines on placenta accreta spectrum disorders: Epidemiology. Int J Gynaecol Obstet. 2018 Mar; 140(3): 265-273.

[21] Say L, Chou D, Gemmill A, Tunçalp Ö, Moller AB, Daniels J, Gülmezoglu AM, Temmerman M, Alkema L. Global causes of maternal death: a WHO systematic analysis. Lancet Glob Health. 2014 Jun;2(6):e323-33. doi: 10.1016/S2214-109X(14)70227-X. Epub 2014 May 5. PMID: 25103301

[22] Dehury RK, Samal J. Maternal Health Situation in Bihar and Madhya Pradesh: A Comparative Analysis of State Fact Sheets of National Family Health Survey (NFHS)-3 and 4. J ClinDiagn Res. 2016 Sep; 10(9):IE01-IE04. doi: 10.7860/JCDR/2016/19079.8404. Epub 2016 Sep 1. PMID: 27790466; PMCID: PMC50 71966.

[23] Institute of Medicine (US) Committee on Improving Birth Outcomes. Improving Birth Outcomes: Meeting the Challenge in the Developing World. Bale JR, Stoll BJ, Lucas AO, editors. Washington (DC): National Academies Press (US); 2003. PMID: 25057689

[24] Kohli C, Kishore J, Sharma S, Nayak H. Knowledge and practice of Accredited Social Health Activists for maternal healthcare delivery in Delhi. J Family Med Prim Care. 2015 Jul-Sep;4(3):359-63. doi: 10.4103/2249-4863.161317. PMID: 26288774; PMCID: PMC4535095

[25] Rchiips.org. 2020. Available from: http://rchiips.org/pdf/state/Maharashtra.pdf

[26] http://nrhmorissa.gov.in/

[27] http://www.sihfw.nrhmharyana.gov.in/

[28] https://www.who.int/reproductivehealth/publications/maternal_perinatal_health/peripartum-infections-guidelines/en/

Chapter 5

Challenges in the Delivery Room: Integrated Analysis of Biomarkers Predicting Complications in Lupus Pregnancy

Eugen Ancuta, Dragos Valentin Crauciuc, Emil Anton, Carmen Anton, Eduard Crauciuc, Dumitru Sofroni, Larisa Sofroni, Claudia Mihailov and Codrina Ancuta

Abstract

Pregnancy in autoimmune rheumatic diseases remains a real challenge in clinical practice due to complex interplay between disease activity, pregnancy and drugs, and account for potential influence of pregnancy on rheumatic condition and the impact of disease on pregnancy outcomes. Indeed, innovative and successful therapies have dramatically improved the quality of life in immune-mediated rheumatic conditions and, subsequently, allowed more patients of reproductive age to plan a pregnancy/to conceive. The purpose of this chapter is to discuss emerging data about the interaction of pregnancy and systemic erythematosus lupus (SLE) focusing on modulation of the immune system by pregnancy, pregnancy outcomes in women with active lupus, biomarkers of adverse pregnancy outcomes (APO) including predictors of pre-eclampsia, predictors of obstetric complications in SLE, the influence of autoantibodies on fetal health, and, finally, evidence about rheumatologic and obstetric follow-up. There are still unmet needs in this new field of reproductive rheumatology and it becomes crucial that researchers, physicians (rheumatologists, specialists in maternofetal medicine, obstetricians) and midwifes share their knowledge and expertise in counseling women with SLE wishing to conceive, assisting pregnancy and managing different issues related to APO as well as drug optimization in preconception, during pregnancy and postpartum period.

Keywords: midwife, systemic lupus erythematosus, pregnancy

1. Introduction

While documenting the role of midwifery in medical education, it is important to understand how rheumatic diseases respond to pregnancy and to allow continued development of multidisciplinary models in order to facilitate all reasonable steps in reproduction with the best available scientific evidence for health professionals.

In fact, a detailed introspection is pivotal to understand the relationship between the perception of pain, mental stress and/or physical injuries during active labor, midwife confidence and ability to handle labor.

Besides, labor quality cannot be defined by only two or three parameters; therefore, companies should consider knowledge capacities and not price whenever they decide to invest in delivery quality. These comments raise added question: "Is effort better spent at the national level to encourage labor or support for women and their babies during pregnancy?" We are optimistic about Romanian institutions supporting educational efforts that contribute to an adequate quality of labor.

Midwifes are far more important for parturient life providing optimal care based on monitoring of fetal heart, recording delivery data as well as communication with giving birth women [1–4]; also, they will provide our students clear targets for their educational and self-improvement goals.

In fact, it is well known that midwifes give support to the following events: monitor and examine women during pregnancy, breast-feeding and bathing, assist mother during labor, offer advices about still-birth, neonatal abnormality or neonatal death, make referrals to doctors, screening tests in hospital, participate in the training and supervision of youngers colleagues and students [1–4].

Continuous presence of midwifes on bed-side of parturient had positive effects, comprising a decreased risk of hemorrhage and transfusion, a decrease in urinary incontinence, reducing the delivery duration and other complications [1–4].

Pregnancy in women with immune-mediated rheumatic diseases (IMRDs) such as rheumatoid arthritis, connective tissue disorders (lupus and scleroderma), juvenile idiopathic arthritis and spondyloarthropathies is still considered a challenge in routine practice given the complex changes in the maternal immune response and the interferences between disease, pregnancy and medication [4–10].

Systemic lupus erythematosus (SLE) is commonly defined by higher maternal and fetal risk compared with pregnancy in general population, meaning that pregnant lupus patients present worse maternal as well as fetal outcomes including increased the risk of abortion, (pre)-eclampsia and placental complications [4–10].

Recent studies have shown that pregnant women with confirmed diagnosis of SLE are more likely to have hypertension, renal disease, diabetes, cerebrovascular disease, thyroid disorders, ischemic heart disease, pregnancy induced hypertension, preterm delivery, emergent caesarian sections, small for gestational age, congenital anomalies [4–11].

Clinical and/or subclinical inflammation, autoantibodies profile, hormonal dysfunction and immune abnormalities related to lupus may unquestionably contribute to pregnancy complications [5–10].

Furthermore, physiologic changes related to pregnancy are difficult to distinguish not only from disease-related manifestations but also from disease exacerbations, requiring a multidisciplinary approach with close rheumatic, obstetrical, and neonatal monitoring in order to optimize both maternal and fetal outcomes [5–10].

Although several biomarkers predicting complications in early pregnancy have already been investigated, preconception assessment is mandatory to stratify the risk in such patients. In addition to routine pregnancy labs, specific assessments should be reviewed during pregnancy comprising immune profile (total antinuclear antibodies, anti-double stranded DNA antibodies, antiphospholipid antibodies, complement level), inflammatory tests (erythrocyte sedimentation rate, C reactive protein) and proteinuria [5–10].

This review outlines detailed requirements during pre-pregnancy, pregnancy and early motherhood of reproductive-aged women diagnosed with autoimmune rheumatic diseases. We will discuss the major risks associated with pregnancy in SLE as well as management recommendations and we will focus on challenges in the delivery room by integrating the role of biomarkers to predict complications in lupus pregnancy and to foster the responsibility of midwife at parturient bed-side.

2. Healthy pregnancy *vs*. lupus pregnancy

It is critical to mention that pregnancy represents a unique clinical situation, physiologically characterized by a well-documented Th2-cell polarization at both systemic and maternal-fetal interfaces, developed on a background of depressed cellular-mediated immunity, changes in Th1/Th2 cytokine profile, and placental synthesis of complement inhibitors [4, 9, 10]. Also, progressively increased levels of sex hormones - estrogens, progesterone, prolactin, as well as and glucocorticoids are commonly reported during pregnancy [1, 4, 9, 10]. Complex immunological and hormonal adaptive mechanisms are activated to allow the tolerance of fetus classically considered as an immunogenic allograft [4, 9].

A closer look to the pathogenic pathways of autoimmune rheumatic conditions emphasizes specific genetic susceptibility and aberrant immune response driving definite behavior during pregnancy [4, 10]. Rheumatic diseases respond differently to pregnancy, as immune system adjustments may positively or negatively interrelate with underlying autoimmune disease: spontaneous improvement occurs in some of them, while persistent activity or severe flares are seen in others, such as systemic lupus erythematosus [1, 4, 10].

Despite significant progress in understanding and treating autoimmune rheumatic conditions, pregnancy in such patients remains a challenge due to complex interplay between pregnancy, disease activity and medication; the main debate focuses on the paradigm "flare without medication" *vs*. "safe drug in pregnancy", emerging the unmet needs for pregnant rheumatic patients [1, 4, 6, 9, 10].

Furthermore, it is widely recognized that the management of reproductive issues in patients with rheumatic diseases commonly differs from general population, requiring a cross-over team with rheumatologists, specialists in the fields of obstetrics-gynecology and maternal-fetal medicine, and, in special cases, reproductive endocrinology and infertility [1–4, 10]. Patients should be counseled about contraception, pregnancy and lactation; additionally, pregnancy in IMRDs needs to be planned and risks assessed in mother and child [1–4, 10, 11]. High-risk pregnancies require careful monitoring and tailored therapy to secure maternal health and positive pregnancy outcomes [4, 10].

Systemic lupus erythematosus is a multi-system autoimmune disease of still unknown etiology, defined by a wide spectrum of organ involvement occurring on a background of fatigue, fever, joint pain and weight changes, and a chronic evolution with exacerbations alternating with quiescent disease [1, 4, 6, 8]. It develops predominantly in women of their reproductive age, making pregnancy a major concern in routine practice; lupus women have higher risk for infertility, miscarriages, and other pregnancy complications due to disease activity, renal involvement, medications (e.g. cyclophosphamide), and presence of certain autoantibodies (anti- Ro/SSA, anti-La/SSB, antiphospholipid antibodies) [4, 10, 12].

The outcomes of lupus pregnancies have dramatically improved over the last decade thanks to advance understanding of disease and its effects in the body, pregnancy planning, multidisciplinary management and close monitoring [1–6]. However, there are clear differences between pregnancy in general population and lupus pregnancy. While a healthy pregnancy is widely defined by specific immunological and hormonal changes, underlying lupus pregnancy is characterized by higher serum pro-inflammatory cytokines, lesser Th2 polarization, lower estrogen and progesterone levels, lower number of T-Reg defective cells, blockade of complement inhibitors by anti-phospholipid antibodies (aPL), increased placental complement component deposition, aberrant activation and, finally, local inflammation. In another words, we talk about an altered physiological response, leading to significant pregnancy morbidity in lupus patients [1–4, 10].

Furthermore, the physiological modulation of the immune system by pregnancy and related hormonal changes may interact with disease activity in autoimmune rheumatic disorders and drive complications (e.g. disease flares); on the other hand, lupus may have a significant impact on pregnancy outcomes [1, 2, 4, 10]. Disease activity, severity of organ damage, antibody profile and drug treatment may promote maternal (e.g. preeclampsia) and fetal complications (pregnancy loss, intra-uterine growth retardation, preterm birth, even neonatal lupus) [1, 4, 9, 10].

Pregnancy in lupus is still considered at increased risk for adverse pregnancy outcomes (APOs) [1–10]. Pregnant SLE-women can develop in 19–57% cases severe obstetric complications including spontaneous abortion (SA), preeclampsia (PE), intrauterine growth restriction (IUGR), small for gestational age (SGA), preterm birth, fetal death in utero and neonatal death. APOs particularly develop if significantly longer disease duration and higher disease activity 6 preconceptual months, during pregnancy and 6 months postpartum period [1, 4, 9, 10, 12, 13]; furthermore, active SLE at the time of conception is a strong predictor of APOs and current recommendations consider disease quiescence for 6 months prior to conception [1, 4, 10, 12, 13].

A detailed look to one of the most important multiethnic cohort of lupus patients in the PROMISSE (*Predictors of Pregnancy Outcome: Biomarkers in Antiphospholipid Antibody Syndrome and Systemic Lupus Erythematosus*) prospective study revealed APOs in 19% of pregnancies, with fetal and neonatal death in 4% and 1%, respectively, preterm delivery in 9%, and small-for-gestational-age neonate in 10% suggesting how important is to accurately identify, counsel, and manage lupus patients in order to optimize their pregnancy outcomes [1, 14–17].

3. Biomarkers in lupus pregnancy

A *biomarker* is an indicator of normal biological processes, pathogenic processes or responses to an intervention [16]. Besides their triple diagnostic, prognostic and therapeutic value, biomarkers have major implications in personalized medicine [1, 2, 4, 16].

Specific biomarkers and novel serum or urine biomarkers may represent the best choice to classify stage and treat patients with SLE; an extended list includes complement level, specific antibodies level, CXCL10, Galectin 9, SIGLEC-1, IL-1 family, BAFF family, lymphocyte populations as serum biomarkers, as well as urine biomarkers [16].

In an attempt to identify biomarkers in lupus pregnancy, pivotal studies suggested that active disease, prior nephritis, use of antihypertensive medications, antiphospholipid antibodies (aPL), hypocomplementemia and anti-double stranded DNA (anti-dsDNA) antibodies are highly associated with APOs [1, 4, 9, 10].

We will further focus on different APOs in lupus, emphasizing the role of biomarkers in stratifying risks and, eventually, driving a more personalized approach in lupus pregnancy.

3.1 Impact of pregnancy on SLE

3.1.1 Lupus flares associated with pregnancy

It is well known that 40 to 60% of women with SLE will experience a flare during pregnancy or the first post-partum year; moreover, disease can exacerbate at any time during pregnancy and postpartum period, without any clear pattern [1, 2, 4–6, 8]. Commonly utilized instruments to asses disease activity in non-pregnant lupus patients have been specifically adapted and validated for the use in pregnant women [5, 6, 8, 18–20]; *SLE Disease Activity Index in Pregnancy* (SLEPDAI), *modified-SLE Activity Measure for Pregnancy* (m-SLAM) and *Lupus Activity Index in Pregnancy* (LAI-P) and are able to detect changes in disease activity in pregnancy, to monitor and to diagnose flares of maternal disease during gravidity, without mistaking signs and symptoms physiologically associated with pregnancy [1, 4, 5, 8, 18, 21].

According to their severity, lupus flares may be classified as *mild flares* (involving skin and joints), with no major impact on pregnancy outcomes, and *severe flares* (in which kidney features, significant hematologic, serositis and severe arthritis may develop) with poor pregnancy outcomes [1, 2, 5, 6, 8].

Most of lupus exacerbations during pregnancy and postpartum period had mucocutaneous, renal and hematological involvement; additionally, postpartum 6-month period appears to have the highest risk for disease exacerbation and up to 50% of flares in postpartum are severe according to a recent analysis [1, 4–8, 10, 13].

SLE flares critically depend on disease activity 6 to 12 months prior to the conception suggesting that pregnancy outcomes are optimal when disease is in complete clinical remission for 6–12 months before conception; besides, there is a 2 to 4 times risk of flare if active lupus before pregnancy, and a SLEDAI≥4 points 6 months before pregnancy and lupus nephritis are main predictors of adverse maternal outcomes [1, 4–8].

Several factors should be considered for risk stratification in SLE women in preconception [1, 4–10] (**Table 1**).

Biomarkers predicting lupus flare in pregnancy may be classified in three main categories, as follows [1, 4–8, 10]:

- *predictors of poor pregnancy outcomes,* including active maternal disease, any prior or current renal involvement, specific autoantibody subsets and advanced organ damage;

- *predictors for SLE flares during pregnancy,* such as increased SLE activity in the 3 to 6 months before conception, discontinuation of specific medication (hydroxychloroquine) during pregnancy, history of frequent and significant flares, low C4 levels at preconception visit; and

- *predictors of renal flare during pregnancy,* including serum creatinine>1.2 mg/dL, proteinuria>500 mg/24 hours at the time of conception and low C4 serum levels, but not low C3 or dsDNA levels.

Although it is widely recognized that low C3 and C4 levels are associated with active SLE, it seems that low complement occurring during SLE pregnancy may predict APOs [1, 4, 6–8, 22]. Recent data confirm that low C4 at preconception predict flares during pregnancy and suggest that complement evaluation during pregnancy is suitable to detect the high-risk patients that require a more vigilant SLE monitoring and management [23]. Surprisingly, the same study failed to demonstrate any statistical correlation between lupus flare and anti-dsDNA positivity, disease activity (SLEDAI at preconception visit and SLEPDAI during pregnancy), antiphospholipid antibodies positivity as well as clinical SLE manifestations [1, 4–8, 18, 24].

SLE specific risk factors	General risk factors
• active SLE	• maternal age,
• serological activity	• arterial hypertension
• lupus nephritis	• diabetes mellitus
• anti-Ro/SSA and anti-La/SSB antibodies	• overweight/obesity
• anti-phospholipid antibodies	• smoking
• antiphospholipid syndrome	• alcohol use
• organ damage	• thyroid disease

Table 1.
Risk stratification of SLE in preconception period.

	Lupus flare/ activity	Normal pregnancy that can mimic a lupus flare
Clinical	Active malar rash Oral/nasal ulcers Inflammatory arthritis Lymphadenopathy Fever >38 without infection Serositis	Palmar and facial erythema Arthralgia/ joint effusion Fatigue Hair loss Mild edema Mild dyspnea
Labs	Increased ESR Anemia (<10.5 g/dl) Thrombocytopenia, leukopenia, lymphopenia ≥ 25% complement drop dsDNA rising Hematuria or cellular casts Proteinuria ≥300 mg/dL	Increased ESR Anemia due to hemodilution Mild thrombocytopenia Increase in complement dsDNA stable Rare hematuria Proteinuria <300 mg/dL

ESR, Erythrocyte sedimentation rate; dsDNA, double stranded DNA.

Table 2.
Differences between lupus flare and physiological pregnancy changes.

On the other hand, many authors reported that disease activity during pregnancy increases the risk of APO, while patients with sustained low lupus disease activity scores have significantly lower APO rates [8, 13, 18].

Recognizing a lupus flare can be difficult given that normal changes related to pregnancy can mimic lupus activity [1, 4, 10]. Main clinical and lab assessment in lupus flare and normal pregnancy are summarized in table above (**Table 2**).

Serological biomarkers are suitable for monitoring lupus activity, but serological activity that develops during pregnancy, especially in the context of clinical activity, may be associated with increased risk for pregnancy loss, intrauterine growth restriction and preterm birth [1, 4–10].

Finally, the so-called *'critical' clinical and serological lupus phenotypes* define patients at increased risk for pregnancy complications; such phenotypes require a special monitoring during pregnancy and encompass for past or present history of lupus nephritis, anti-Ro/SSA and/or La/SSB positivity and aPL positivity or SLE associated with APS [1, 4–10].

3.1.2 Lupus nephritis and pregnancy

It is basically recognized that renal activity may be associated with APOs, requiring a strict follow-up based on urine protein excretion, urine sediment analysis (haematuria, urinary casts) as well as serum creatinine level and glomerular filtration rate [1, 2, 4–9]. Moreover, urinary levels of CXCL10, and CXCL16 are highly increased in lupus nephritis, TCD4 cells may be an indicator of all treatment response and CCL2 sensitive indicator of renal flare [16].

Recommendations for the approach of pregnancy in the context of lupus nephritis have been released by *European League Against Rheumatism* (EULAR) in 2017. Severe renal flares during pregnancy not responding to drugs with an acceptable safety profile (azathioprine, antimalarials) warrant for a complex, multidisciplinary management, with potential early termination of pregnancy and/or use of embryotoxic drugs if required. [4, 6–8, 25–28].

Several practical points should be emphasized as follows:

- high SLE activity has critical, unfavorable effect on pregnancy;
- a high activity score SLEDAI≥4 out of 105 in the 6 months before conception raises the flare rate;
- renal flares usually occur if pre-existing renal involvement, particularly if remission was not achieved before pregnancy;
- the timing of flare is unpredictable, regular monitoring being indicated during pregnancy and postpartum;
- antimalarials should not be discontinued during pregnancy even in lupus remission [1, 4, 6, 8, 10].

3.2 Impact of SLE on pregnancy

3.2.1 Pre-eclampsia (PE)

Considered as a syndrome unique to pregnancy, preeclampsia remains a significant maternal complication in lupus pregnancy [1, 4–10] and a challenge in clinical practice. Key parameters that allow us to distinguish between PE and SLE activity are listed below (**Table 3**) [1, 4–8, 10, 22, 29]. Interestingly, serologic biomarkers can also distinguish between SLE flare (decreased serum C3 and C4 levels associated with increased anti-dsDNA concentrations) and pre-eclampsia. [4, 7, 8, 22, 24].

Mild PE refers to the new onset of hypertension (≥140/90 mmHg) associated with proteinuria (≥300 mg/24 h urine specimen) after 20 weeks of gestation in a previously normotensive women, while *severe PE* account for new onset proteinuric hypertension and at least one of the following: thrombocytopenia (less than 100.000 platelets/mm^3), symptoms of central nervous system dysfunction, proteinuria ≥5 g/24 h and oliguria, liver involvement (serum transaminase at least twice normal), severe blood pressure elevation (≥160/110 mmHg). It is undoubtedly associated with high risk for stroke, preterm birth, death and eclampsia [1, 4, 10].

Furthermore, preeclampsia should also be differentiated by active lupus nephritis and there are several clinical and lab parameters that help to correctly assess the patient and recognize the renal involvement or pregnancy complication (**Table 4**) [1, 4, 10].

Finally, biomarkers predicting preeclampsia in lupus are already documented, as follows [4, 8, 22, 29, 30]:

- *SLE-specific factors* - active lupus nephritis (especially class III or IV), renal failure at the time of conception, sustained use of prednisone (≥ 20 mg/day during pregnancy), thrombocytopenia, active SLE at conception, low C4, anti-RNP positivity, presence of aPL antibodies; and

- *Maternal factors* - age ≥ 40 years, previous personal or family history of preeclampsia, pre-existing hypertension or diabetes, multiple pregnancies, obesity, low pro-angiogenic factors (VEGF, PIGF1), high anti-angiogenic factors (sFlt-1, soluble endoglin), increased vascular resistance in uterine artery with deficient spiral artery remodeling.

The use of vascular endothelial growth factor (VEGF), placental growth factor (PlGF) and FMS–like tyrosine kinase-1(sFlt-1) are useful for the differential diagnosis between nephritis and preeclampsia [1, 4, 10].

Asymptomatic aPL-positive patients (without any pregnancy complications or history of thrombosis) are not generally treated with prophylactic therapy to prevent pregnancy loss. However, presence of aPL regardless of clinical history is considered a risk factor for development of preeclampsia [4, 5, 8, 10, 22, 29].

Although the outcomes of lupus pregnancy have dramatically improved, *pregnancy loss, preterm birth, low birth weight and cesarean section* are still reported in such patient population [1, 4, 9, 10].

3.2.2 Pregnancy loss (PL)

Pregnancy loss has decreased from 45% in the '60s to a 20–33% nowadays, but we can still talk about fewer than expected children in SLE due to recurrent miscarriage, fetal loss, stillbirth and increased perinatal death [1, 4, 10].

Main causes for pregnancy loss are increased complement activation and placental inflammation (C5a), secondary antiphospholipid syndrome (APS) with specific aPL antibodies, complete atrio-ventricular block (CHB) secondary to anti-Ro/SSA and La/SSB antibodies (diagnosis before gestational week 20 increases four times the intrauterine mortality rate), ventricular rate 50–59 bpm (with a five times higher mortality rate if under 50 pm) [1, 4, 10].

	Preeclampsia	**SLE activity**
Risk factors		
1st pregnancy	Increased risk	No impact
Preeclampsia in prior pregnancy	Increased risk	No impact
Multifetal pregnancy	Increased risk	Unknown impact
History of LN	Increased risk	Increased risk
Timing in pregnancy	Always >20 weeks, usually >30 weeks	Any time in pregnancy
Laboratory findings		
Active urine sediment	Usually, negative	Positive
Coombs test	Usually, negative	May be positive
Anti-platelet antibody	Usually, negative	May be positive
C3 and C4	Usually, normal	Decreased
Anti-dsDNA ab	Normal or stable	High
Serum uric acid	>5.5 mg/dL	No change
Urine calcium	Low	Normal
Proteinuria	High, even>5 g/24 h	Present ++
Serum creatinine	High	Normal or high
Physical findings		
Dermatologic disease*	Not present	Present
Arthritis	Not present	Present
Serositis	Not present	Present
Blood pressure	High ≥160/110 mmHg	Normal or high

**Vasculitis, Discoid rash, Mouth ulcers, Alopecia.*

Table 3.
Differences between preeclampsia and SLE activity.

Clinical & labs	Active lupus nephritis	Preeclampsia
Hypertension	Onset before 20 weeks	Onset after 20 weeks
24 h Proteinuria	Usually high (≥ 300 mg/day)	Usually high (≥ 300 mg/day)
Urinary sediment	Active	Inactive
Uric acid	Usually≤5.5 mg/dL, but may be increased	Usually hyperuricemia (> 5.5 mg/dL)
DNA antibody level	Usually positive or rising	Stable or negative
24 h urine calcium	≥ 195 mg/day	< 195 mg/day
Complement levels	Usually low or decreasing (≥ 25% drop)	Usually high or stable (normal)
Clinical lupus symptoms (arthritis, rash, fever)	Often present	Usually absent

Table 4.
Differentiation of active lupus nephritis from preeclampsia (adapted [10]).

Four main types of pregnancy loss predictors have been so far identified, as follows:

- *disease activity,* meaning active SLE 6 months prior to conception and active SLE during pregnancy;
- *secondary APS,* with either single, dual or multiple positivity for aPL; triple positivity is not better than lupus anticoagulant alone in predicting adverse pregnancy outcomes;
- *organ involvement - nephritis,* comprising preexisting lupus nephritis and first trimester proteinuria (active lupus nephritis particularly class III and IV), thrombocytopenia, chronic hypertension and prior pregnancy loss; and
- *lupus serology* with low C3 and C4 serum levels and anti-dsDNA antibodies [1, 2, 4–6, 10].

3.2.3 Preterm birth (PTB)

Preterm birth meaning pregnancy termination under 37 weeks of gestation is still reported in up to 40% of lupus pregnancies; even women with quiescent lupus prior to and during pregnancy have a higher rate of preterm delivery, with delayed development and lung immaturity, poor long-term outcomes and prolonged hospitalization (if PTB under 30 weeks) as main consequences [1, 2, 4–6, 9, 10].

Spontaneous or lupus-related PTB reflects hormonal dysfunction as well as clinical and subclinical inflammation: activation of maternal or fetal hypo-thalamus pituitary axis with cortisol and prostaglandin production, poor placental development with lower estradiol levels, inflammation with CK, prostaglandin and complement activation.

Conversely *induced PTB* mirrors high rates medical complications in women with lupus and may be related to disease activity, prior and current lupus nephritis, renal failure, maternal hypertension, lupus anticoagulant and corticosteroids use [1, 4, 6, 9, 10].

Several predictors of preterm birth in lupus pregnancy have already been reported, including:

- *predictors for spontaneous PTB*, such as low estradiol at mid-gestation (marker of poor placenta function), high ferritin at mid gestation (marker of inflammation), high uric acid at mid gestation (marker of poor kidney function), oral prednisone, elevated anti-dsDNA, low complement; and
- *predictors for induced PTB*, such as lupus activity during pregnancy, prior lupus nephritis, active lupus nephritis during the first trimester, renal insufficiency, lupus anticoagulant, hypertension, as well as glucocorticoids [1, 4, 10].

3.2.4 Intrauterine growth restriction (IUGR)

Defined as a condition in which the fetus is smaller than expected for the number of weeks of pregnancy, the three different types of IUGR (*type I symmetric or primary,* 20–25% of cases*; type II asymmetric or secondary; type III or intermediate IUGR*) may depend on poor placentation and endothelial dysfunction, persistent inflammation (clinical, subclinical), high autoantibodies levels and medication (excess glucocorticoids have impact on placenta vascular resistance and fetal growth).

IUGR is significantly increased in SLE pregnancy (about 30%) and is typically associated with increased risk of perinatal morbidity and mortality as well as short and long-term neurological complications [1, 2, 4, 9, 10].

Predictors of IUGR include changes in cerebral brain blood perfusion (Doppler), increase in circulating mitochondrial DNA content, maternal hypertension, APS and active lupus [1, 2, 4, 10].

Interesting data are reported during the PROMISSE study - *Predictors of Pregnancy Outcome: Bio-Markers In antiphospholipid antibody Syndrome and Systemic Lupus Erythematosus*: up to 80% of lupus patients had a favorable pregnancy outcome. *Poor outcome predictors* recognized in PROMISE study are increase in lupus activity during pregnancy (SLEPDAI) $\geq$4 at baseline increase over baseline in SLEPDAI $\geq$3 at 20 or 32 weeks, high titer of aPL and high median uric acid levels at baseline, high prolactin levels related to disease activity and poor fetal outcome; SLE patients without anti-PRL antibodies had a significantly higher frequency of maternal and fetal complications, as premature deliveries or IUGR [1, 4, 5, 14–18].

3.2.5 Neonatal lupus (NLE)

Considered as fetal manifestation of passively acquired autoimmunity, neonatal lupus is caused by or associated with maternal anti-Ro/SSA (52 or 60KDa) and/or, rarely, anti-La/SSB (48KDa) positivity; around 10% cases present with skin rash, 20% with transient cytopenia, and up to one third with mild transient high levels of transaminases; all of these complications are usually short-lived and spontaneously resolves as the child's maternal antibodies disappear [1, 2, 4, 10]. More severe is the complete (third-degree) heart block (CBH) that occurs rarely, in about 2% of pregnancies of women with anti-Ro/La positivity who had never a prior infant with NLE; however, the rate increases up to 18% if a history of prior infant who had either cutaneous or cardiac NLE [1, 2, 4, 10].

The impact of autoantibodies on fetal health was analyzed in different cohorts, suggesting their role as predictors for NLE and CBH [1, 2, 4, 10]. High titers of antibodies carry on a specific risk for CBH. Regarded as a major and irreversible complication, CBH may associate with fatal outcome in one out of five cases (*in utero* or death first year of life), while more than half require a pacemaker [1, 4, 10].

Absolute contraindications	Relative contraindications
Severe organ damage • severe pulmonary hypertension (systolic PAP > 50 mmHg or symptomatic) • severe restrictive lung disease (forced vital capacity FVC < 1 L) • advanced heart failure • previous severe preeclampsia • HELLP syndrome despite therapy • advanced renal failure (creatinine>2.8 mg/dL)	• severe lupus flare within the past 6 months • active lupus nephritis within the past 6 months • stroke within the previous 6 months • teratogenic drugs 6 months prior to the current pregnancy

Table 5.
Contraindication for pregnancy in SLE.

3.3 Contraindications for pregnancy in SLE

Absolute pregnancy and relative contraindications in SLE are listed above (**Table 5**) [1, 4, 9, 10].

3.4 Predicting outcomes in lupus pregnancy

Since SLE is highly associated with poor obstetric outcomes, predicting the risks is critical for optimizing pregnancy success [4, 10]. The risk of undesirable fetal outcomes estimation in the early first trimester of pregnancy by rheumatologists may guarantee a desirable pregnancy outcome [4, 10, 31].

An clinical decision support system has already been developed in SLE pregnant women based on the artificial neural network (multi-layer perceptron machine-learning algorithm, MPL) by Khadijeh and colab. (2017) helping physician to predict the pregnancy outcomes in women with SLE based on 16 different features (https://pubmed.ncbi.nlm.nih.gov/27919382/) [31].

Cumulative clinical, laboratory and serological parameters have been tested and classified as qualitative and quantitative factors [31].

Distribution of *qualitative features* predicting SLE-pregnancy outcomes and their influence on spontaneous abortion and live births focus on *flare-up* (yes/ no), *anemia and leukopenia before pregnancy* (positive/ negative), *APS* (positive/ negative), *anticardiolipin antibodies IgG in the first trimester of pregnancy* (positive/ negative), *anti-dsDNA in the first trimester of pregnancy* (positive/ negative), C-*reactive protein before pregnancy* (positive/ negative), *azathioprine before or in the first trimester* (use/ non-use) *and aspirin in the first trimester of pregnancy* (use/non-use) [31].

On the other hand, *quantitative features* predicting pregnancy outcome in SLE include *platelets count before and during pregnancy, hematuria during pregnancy, proteinuria before and during pregnancy, C3 complement level before and during pregnancy, and hydroxychloroquine dose before pregnancy* [31].

The use of the above-mentioned factors can help the rheumatologist to predict spontaneous abortion or live birth, allowing the optimal anti-rheumatic treatment [31].

4. Guidelines for the management of pregnant lupus women

Guidelines recommend addressing family planning in women with chronic rheumatic diseases focusing on medication, disease control and reproductive health outcomes [1–8].

The preconception counseling should address several aspects regarding fertility and pregnancy issue in women with SLE especially the impact of pregnancy on disease outcomes and vice-versa the impact of disease and SLE-related medication on maternal and fetal outcomes, factor that can influence the pregnancy course (e.g., maternal age, medication, previous pregnancies) and, finally, the attitude face to an unplanned pregnancy (**Table 6**).

Pregnancy may be responsible for exacerbation of SLE clinical activity and, in turn, active disease may challenge pregnancy course [4]. Since the outcomes of SLE pregnancies and the complication rates are linked to diseases activity, achievement of remission or stable disease is recommended before pregnancy to reduce maternal-fetal problems [1, 4, 10].

Adequate **preconception assessment** should be advanced including a complete obstetric-gynecological history, comorbidities, contraindications and risks of pregnancies based on individual evaluation of clinical SLE activity at the time of conception, antibody panel and medication (**Table 7**).

Apart from this plan before pregnancy, another check list including **risk factors for maternal and fetal complications in SLE pregnancy** should be included in patient's file and updated during pregnancy according to individual data (**Table 8**).

Women with SLE require additional care and will qualify as high-risk pregnancies; they should be informed about specific risks such as IUGR, pregnancy loss, preterm birth and neonatal lupus [4, 10]. High risk lupus pregnancy factors comprise active lupus, medication that can cause birth defects and untreated antiphospholipid syndrome.

Gestational planning and the follow-up should be performed by a multidisciplinary team including at least an experienced in high-risk pregnancy obstetrician and treating rheumatologist with broad experience in planning and control pregnancy in SLE; accurate obstetric visits as well as strict control of the underlying lupus are essential, but the schedule of follow-ups will depend on both obstetric evaluation and disease activity [1, 4–6, 10].

Thus, we can identify at least three situations [4]:

- *pregnant SLE in remission or low disease activity, with a clinically stable disease;* in such patients, follow-up visits will be planned every 4 to 6 weeks during the first two trimesters and on a basis of 2 weeks between 32 weeks of gestation to the end of pregnancy;

- *pregnant SLE women with SLE exacerbation and/or developing obstetric complications*; follow-ups will be scheduled every 4 weeks by the obstetrician and every 4 to 6 weeks by the rheumatologist until the 20th week of gestation, every 2 weeks between 21st and 28th week, and weekly until the end of pregnancy;

- *pregnant SLE with anti-Ro/La positivity* will undergo weekly fetal echocardiography (PR interval, fetal heart rate) between 16th and 26th week of gestation.

Check-ups visits include preplanned evaluation tests [4]:

- *at each visit* - monitoring blood pressure, body weight and basic physical examination, urinalysis as well as complement and anti-dsDNA antibodies;

- *at 8–12 weeks*: complete blood count, erythrocyte sedimentation rate, C reactive protein, routine glucose, renal and liver function; in the case of a SLE flare, blood samples should be performed more frequently;

Preconception issue
Impact of SLE on fertility
Impact of SLE on pregnancy
Impact of pregnancy on SLE
Planning the pregnancy: disease activity prior conception, drug modification prior to conception, calendar for visits, pre-pregnancy tests
Measures required during pregnancy and breastfeeding
Risks in newborn: risks to develop maternal disease, sequelae related to medication used during pregnancy, special care
Unforeseen management of pregnancy

Table 6.
Preconception counseling in SLE women (adapted [4]).

Preconception steps
1. Make a complete obstetric-gynecological history • Fertility issues • Data about previous pregnancies: parity, term delivery, type of delivery (vaginal/ caesarian section), abortions, fetal loss • Complications: preeclampsia, HELLP, hypertension, thrombosis • IUGR, low birth weight
2. Make a list of relevant comorbidities • Hypertension, diabetes
3. Assess SLE activity, organ damage, history of flares • Activity scores (SLEDAI, SLAM, LAI), damage scores (SLICC/ ACR) • Last flare (time, duration, medication) • Remission/ sustained remission; low disease activity/ high disease activity; stable disease
4. Evaluate treatment plan and reevaluate therapeutic options • Glucocorticoids, antimalarials, immunosuppressives, biological agents during the last 6–12 months • Contraindicated drugs in pregnancy and time to last administration • Adapt medication according to disease activity
5. Identify contraindications for pregnancy (absolute and relative contraindications that require postponed pregnancy)
6. Estimate maternal and fetal risk during pregnancy • Complication in previous pregnancies • Age, disease activity, medication, serology
7. Basic lab tests • Standard analysis • SLE-related: complement, ANA, anti-dsDNA, aPL (lupus anticoagulant, anti-β2 glycoprotein, anticardiolipin), anti-Ro/ La
Conclude on risks, complications, follow-up
• Disease activity • Medication • Risk factor for adverse pregnancy outcomes • Plan of action if maternal or fetal complications

Table 7.
Algorithm for pregnancy planning in SLE women (adapted [4]).

Risk factors
1. Previous adverse obstetric outcomes
• Preeclampsia/ severe preeclampsia
• HELLP syndrome
2. Previous thrombotic events
• Thrombosis 6 months prior to pregnancy
3. Chronic kidney disease
• Creatinine >2.8 mg/dL
4. Risk factors for preeclampsia
• Age > 40
• Family or personal history of preeclampsia
• Multiple pregnancies
• Nulliparity
• Diabetes
• Obesity or hypertension before pregnancy
• Active SLE
• History of lupus nephritis class III or IV
• aPL positivity
5. SLE
• high risk for flare
• history of abortion, neonatal deaths, premature delivery, low birth weights infants
• avoid pregnancy in severe pulmonary hypertension, interstitial lung disease, heart failure, stroke
• avoid pregnancy if severe flare the last 6 months
6. Evidence of APS
• history of abortion, neonatal deaths, premature delivery, low birth weights infants
• avoid pregnancy in severe pulmonary hypertension or thrombosis within the last 6 months

Table 8.
Check list: risk factors for maternal and fetal complication in SLE pregnancy (adapted [4]).

Disease activity should be assessed using indexes adapted for the use during pregnancy (e.g. SLEPDAI), as gravidity may influence certain variables used in the evaluation of activity scores.

Two main recommendations are on the so-called "To do list" for pregnant SLE-women [1–4]:

- see your rheumatologist at least once every trimester;
- see your obstetrician and perinatologist regularly, frequently and tell them about anything new or abnormal in your health.

All the above-mentioned specialists play specific roles in managing the disease and may result in decreased hospital stay and/or serious morbidity and mortality. This can be also largely attributed to the excellent work of midwifes and inter-disciplinary approach on Public Health. Doctors and midwifes collaborate with researches in creating a research group of professionals in order to monitor and evaluate the safety of women giving birth [1–3].

These demonstrated that midwifes support is indispensable for the wellbeing of childbearing women and their infants before and after delivery.

4.1 ACR recommendations for reproductive health-care in SLE

In 2020, *American College of Rheumatology* (ACR) releases an updated guideline with recommendations for reproductive health-care in rheumatic diseases, particularly SLE with and without anti-Ro/La and aPL antibodies [6].

Hereby we summarized the most important statements regarding pregnancy counseling, assessment and monitoring to improve maternal and fetal outcomes in SLE women (**Figure 1**) [6]:

- ACR strongly suggests as standard good practice counseling SLE women who are considering pregnancy and proposing pregnancy in quiescent/low disease activity. Besides, ACR advise maintaining parallel care with specialists in obstetrics-gynecology, maternal-fetal medicine, neonatology [6];

- if lupus woman wishing to conceive is currently on drugs incompatible with pregnancy, ACR strongly recommend switching to a pregnancy-compatible one and observing for sufficient time to assess efficacy and tolerability of the new medication [6];

- moreover, if active lupus that requires medication during pregnancy, ACR strongly recommend initiating or continuing a pregnancy-compatible steroid-sparing medication, as both active disease and continuous high-dose glucocorticoid treatment may account for maternal and fetal harm [6, 31];

- all SLE-women require antimalarials - hydroxychloroquine (HCQ) during pregnancy if possible; if a patient is already taking HCQ, ACR strongly recommend continuing it during pregnancy, but in cases not on HCQ, it is conditionally recommended if no contraindication [6, 31];

- *monitoring SLE activity* with clinical history, examination, and laboratory tests *at least once per trimester* is strongly indicated because active disease may affect both maternal and pregnancy outcomes; thus, although testing for anti-Ro/La once before or early in pregnancy is strongly recommended, given the relative

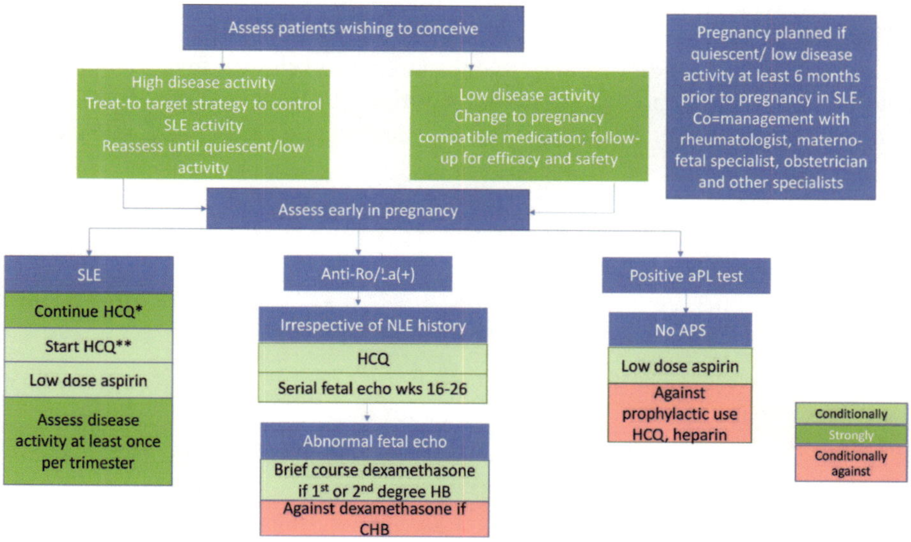

Figure 1.
*Pregnancy counseling, assessment and management in woman with SLE (ACR2020 adapted) [6]. *If on; **if not a contraindication; NLE, neonatal lupus; HB, heart block; CBH, complete heart block.*

persistence of unchanged titers of these antibodies, ACR strongly recommend *against* repeating the test during pregnancy. Besides, it is also strongly recommend testing for aPL before or early in pregnancy, while repeating these tests during pregnancy is not necessary [6];

- in pregnant anti-Ro/LA patient with no history of infants with NLE or CBH, ACR conditionally recommend serial fetal echocardiography (eventually less frequent than weekly, but no interval specified) between 16 to 26 weeks; if a prior infant with NLE or CHB, ACR conditionally recommends strict follow-up using fetal echocardiography weekly, between 16 to 26 weeks [6];

- moreover, all women who are positive for anti-Ro/SSA and/or anti-La/SSB positivity conditionally require with HCQ during pregnancy as there is a lower risk of the current fetus developing CHB under HCQ [6, 32];

- low-dose aspirin (81 or 100, but not more than 150 mg daily) is conditionally recommended in the first trimester; in addition, in pregnant women with positive aPL who do not meet criteria for obstetric or thrombotic APS, ACR conditionally recommend treating with prophylactic aspirin during pregnancy as preeclampsia prophylaxis, beginning early in pregnancy (before 16 weeks) and continuing through delivery [6, 32];

- for pregnant anti-Ro/SSA and/or anti-La/SSB positive patients and fetal first- or second-degree heart block shown on echocardiography, ACR conditionally recommend treatment with oral dexamethasone 4 mg daily; nevertheless, if CHB (without other cardiac inflammation) develop, ACR is conditionally *against* dexamethasone [6, 32].

4.2 EULAR 2020 consensus-based core set data for pregnancy in SLE

In an effort to increase knowledge about pregnancy course and safety of treatment in women with immune mediated rheumatic disorders, *European League Against Rheumatology* published in 2020 its first consensus-based core data set for prospective pregnancy registries in rheumatology [5].

The *EULAR Task Force* recommended disease-specific items, autoantibodies/laboratory markers and disease activity measurements relevant for different IMRDs including SLE. aPL antibodies, particularly anti-cardiolipin, and anti-beta-2-glycoprotein-I antibodies as well as lupus anticoagulant; antinuclear and anti-dsDNA

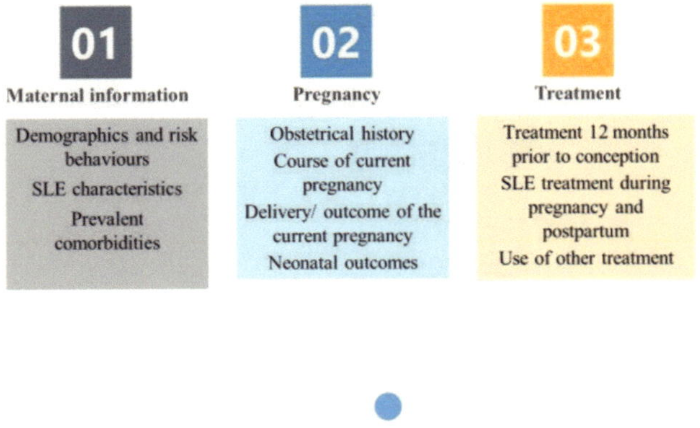

Figure 2.
EULAR core set data for pregnancy in rheumatology (adapted [5]).

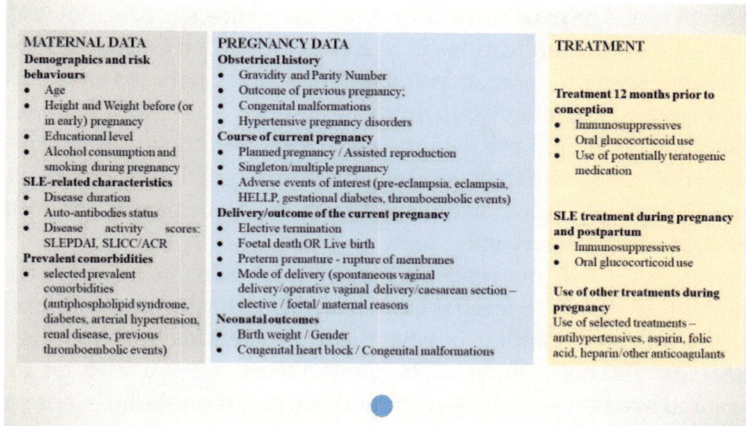

Figure 3.
Proposed core-set data for the midwifery room (adapted from EULAR 2020) [5].

antibodies, extractable nuclear antigen antibodies such as anti-Ro/La, anti-Sm and anti-U1-ribonucleoprotein, but also serum C3 and C4 levels should be collected as recommended by EULAR, while follow-up indexes include SLEPDAI and SLICC/ACR damage index [4, 5, 18].

EULAR endorsed three core set data on clinically relevant parameters - maternal information, pregnancy and treatment [1–3, 5, 21] (**Figure 2**); *maternal information* refers to demographics and risk behaviors, disease characteristics of the underlying SLE and prevalent comorbidities; *pregnancy* data covers obstetrical history, the course, outcomes and delivery of previous and current pregnancy and outcomes of the neonate, while *treatment* domain encompasses for medical treatment within 12 months prior to conception, SLE treatment during pregnancy and postpartum [1–5, 21].

A comprehensive/extensive list of items were considered the most relevant items regarding maternal information and the rheumatic disease as well as pregnancy and neonatal outcomes (**Figure 3**) and should be collected uniformly [1, 3–5, 21].

EULAR endorsed recommendations focused on the time of pregnancy and the 28-day postpartum period (neonatal phase); as the core set represents clinically relevant and feasible parameters, it should be collected once every trimester for the maternal and new-born health evaluation [1, 3, 5, 21].

Besides, as addressing the most important information needed to answer questions about disease activity, medication use and pregnancy outcome, EULAR parameters should be extrapolated, at least in part, for the assessment in daily practice; this will clearly be of help in the midwifery room [1, 3, 5, 21].

5. Conclusion

Reproductive health in SLE remains an important topic as maternal complications and adverse fetal outcomes in lupus still exceed the rate of pregnancy complications in general population. Clinical or subclinical inflammation, autoantibodies, hormonal dysfunction and specific immune alterations of lupus may contribute to pregnancy complications.

Thus, SLE and pregnancy is definitely associated with an increased need for investigations (repeated ultrasound, tests for fetal well-being, predictive biomarkers for pregnancy outcomes) as well as prolonged hospitalization, promoting high prenatal and neonatal burden.

Several biomarkers have been already investigated in early pregnancy and we are now able to predict complications in SLE suggesting that both preconception and follow-up assessments are mandatory to risk-stratify patients and to identity predictors for adverse pregnancy outcomes.

Although pivotal studies have demonstrated a greater rate of caesarian section among lupus pregnancy than in general population, vaginal delivery still remains an option and adequate pelvic assessment should always be performed by midwifes in order to ensure best delivery outcomes.

Moreover, midwifes help our researchers to discover valuable information in an effort of better understand the mechanisms involved in the disease. On the other hand, there is a lack of full understanding of what the researchers in our hospitals are doing, as every researcher and midwife should be allowed to examine patients for any possible medical signs and symptoms and to determine the general status during pregnancy.

This chapter is intended to be a state-of-the-art manuscript focused on improving health-care for pregnant women with SLE.

Conflict of interest

"The authors declare no conflict of interest." or delete this entire section.

Author details

Eugen Ancuta[1], Dragos Valentin Crauciuc[2]*, Emil Anton[2], Carmen Anton[2], Eduard Crauciuc[2], Dumitru Sofroni[3], Larisa Sofroni[4], Claudia Mihailov[5] and Codrina Ancuta[2]

1 "Elena Doamna" Obstetrics and Gynecology Clinical Hospital, Research Department, Iasi, Romania

2 University of Medicine and Pharmacy "Grigore T Popa", Iasi, Romania

3 University of Medicine and Pharmacy "Nicolae Testemitanu", Chisinau, Republic of Moldova

4 Institute of Oncology, Chisinau, Republic of Moldova

5 "Ovidius" University, Constanta, Romania

*Address all correspondence to: crauciuc.dragos@gmail.com

References

[1] Onno Teng YK, Bredewold EOW, Rabelink TJ et al. An evidence-based approach to pre-pregnancy counselling for patients with systemic lupus erythematosus. Rheumatology 2018; 57: 1707-1720. DOI: 10.1093/rheumatology/kex374

[2] Murray K, Moore L, O'Brien C et al. A multidisciplinary approach to reproductive healthcare in women with rheumatic disease. Irish Journal of Medical Science 2020; 189: 237-243; DOI:10.1007/s11845-019-02040-5

[3] Al-Emadi S, Abutiban F, El Zorkany B. Enhancing the care of women with rheumatic diseases during pregnancy: challenges and unmet needs in the Middle East. Clin Rheumatol 2016; 35:25-31. DOI: 10.1007/s10067-015-3052-5

[4] Martínez López JA, García Vivar ML, Cáliz R et al. Recommendations for the evaluation and management of patients with rheumatic autoimmune and inflammatory diseases during the reproductive age, pregnancy, postpartum and breastfeeding. Reumatol Clin 2017; 13:264-281; DOI: 10.1016/j.reuma.2016.05.003

[5] Meissner Y, Fischer-Betz R, Andreoli L, et al. EULAR recommendations for a core data set for pregnancy registries in rheumatology. Ann Rheum Dis 2021; 80:49-56. DOI: 10.1136/annrheumdis-2020-218356

[6] Sammaritano LR, Bermas BL, Chakravarti EE et al, 2020 ACR Guideline for the management of reproductive health in rheumatic and musculoskeletal diseases, Arthritis Care Res (Hoboken) 2020; 72(4):461-488. DOI: 10.1002/acr.24130

[7] Fanouriakis A, Kostopoulou M, Cheema K et al. 2019 Update of the Joint European League Against Rheumatism and European Renal Association–European Dialysis and Transplant Association (EULAR/ERA–EDTA) recommendations for the management of lupus nephritis. Ann Rheum Dis 2020; 79:713-723. DOI: 10.1136/annrheumdis-2020-216924

[8] Andreoli L, Bertsias GK, Agmon-Levin N et al. EULAR recommendations for women's health and the management of family planning, assisted reproduction, pregnancy and menopause in patients with systemic lupus erythematosus and/or antiphospholipid syndrome. Ann Rheum Dis 2017; 76:476-485. DOI: 10.1136/annrheumdis-2016-209770

[9] Østensen M, Brucato A, *et al*. State of the art: reproduction and pregnancy in rheumatic diseases. Autoimmun Rev 2015; 14:376-386. DOI: 10.1016/j.autrev.2014.12.011

[10] Sammaritano LR, Bermas BL. Management of pregnancy and lactation. Best Practice & research. Clinical Rheumatology 2018; 32(6):750-766DOI: 10.1016/j.berh.2019.03.007

[11] Keeling S, Savu A, Kaul P. The impact of SLE on peripartum outcomes: a population level analysis. 27-29 September 2018 B. 10th International Conference on Reproduction, Pregnancy and Rheumatic Diseases; wwwrehumapreg2018.org

[12] Chu J, Sarthak Gupta, Manna Z, et al. Integrating Reproductive Health in SLE in a tertiary care setting (O437); 5-9 November 2020; ACR Convergence 2020; https://meet.acrconvergence.org/meetings/MfEPz5W7ARhiFzkWi

[13] Cetin C, Sivrikpz ST, Tikiz AM, et al. The Correlation Between Pregnancy, Disease Activity and Adverse Pregnancy Outcomes in Patients with Systemic Lupus Erythematosus

(O266); 5-9 November 2020; ACR Convergence 2020;https://meet.acrconvergence.org/meetings/virtual/n6oH2bDqzG3DbKkH2

[14] Yelnik CM, Laskin CA, Porter TF, et al. Lupus anticoagulant is the main predictor of adverse pregnancy outcomes in aPL positive patients: validation of PROMISSE study results. Lupus Science & Medicine 2016;3: e000131. DOI:10.1136/lupus-2015-000131

[15] Buyon J, Kim MY, Guerra MM, et al. Predictors of Pregnancy Outcomes in Patients with Lupus: A Cohort Study. Ann Intern Med 2015;163(3):153-163; DOI: 10.7326/M14-2235.

[16] Capecchi R, Puxeddu I, Pratesi F, Migliorini P. New biomarkers in SLE: from bench to bedside. Rheumatology 2020; 59: v12–v18. DOI:10.1093/rheumatology/keaa484

[17] Salmon JE. PROMISSE: progress in understanding pregnancy complications in patients with SLE. Arthritis Res Ther 2012; 14 (Suppl 3): A39, DOI: 10.1186/ar3973

[18] Andreoli L, Gerardi MC, Fernandes M, *et al*. Disease activity assessment of rheumatic diseases during pregnancy: a comprehensive review of indices used in clinical studies. Autoimmun Rev 2019; 18: 164-176. DOI: 10.1016/j.autrev.2018.08.008

[19] Ruiz-Irastorza G, Khamashta MA, Gordon C, *et al*. Measuring systemic lupus erythematosus activity during pregnancy: validation of the lupus activity index in pregnancy scale. Arthritis Rheum 2004; 51:78-82. DOI:10.1002/art.20081

[20] Yee CS, Akil M, Khamashta M, et al. The BILAG2004-Pregnancy index is reliable for assessment of disease activity in pregnant SLE patients. Rheumatology (Oxford) 2012; 51:1877-1880. DOI:10.1093/rheumatology/kes158

[21] Meissner Y, Strangfeld A, Costedoat-Chalumeau N, *et al*. European Network of Pregnancy Registers in Rheumatology (EuNeP)—an overview of procedures and data collection. Arthritis Res Ther 2019; 21:241. DOI:10.1186/s13075-019-2019-3

[22] Buyon JP, Cronstein BN, Morris M, et al. Serum complement values (C3 and C4) to differentiate between systemic lupus activity and pre-eclampsia. Am J Med 1986; 81:194-200 DOI: 10.1016/0002-9343(86)90251-2.

[23] Crisafulli F, Andreoli L, Filippini M et al. SLE pregnancies: C4 as a predictor of flares and adverse pregnancy outcomes (0262); 5-9 November 2020; ACR Convergence 2020; https://meet.acrconvergence.org/meetings/virtual/LyQKxDtQjH5amXWoF

[24] Clowse ME, Magder LS, Petri M. The clinical utility of measuring complement and anti-dsDNA antibodies during pregnancy in patients with systemic lupus erythematosus. J Rheumatol 2011; **38**:1012-1016. DOI: 10.3899/jrheum.100746

[25] Bramham K, Hunt BJ, Bewley S, *et al.* Pregnancy outcomes in systemic lupus erythematosus with and without previous nephritis. J Rheumatol 2011; **38**:1906-1913. DOI: 10.3899/jrheum.100997

[26] Fischer-Betz R, Specker C, Brinks R, *et al*. Low risk of renal flares and negative outcomes in women with lupus nephritis Conceiving after switching from mycophenolate mofetil to azathioprine. Rheumatology 2013; **52**:1070-1076. DOI: 10.1093/rheumatology/kes425

[27] Koh JH, Ko HS, Lee J, *et al*. Pregnancy and patients with preexisting lupus nephritis: 15 years of

experience at a single center in Korea. Lupus 2015; **24**:764-772. DOI: 10.1177/0961203315572715

[28] Imbasciati E, Tincani A, Gregorini G, et al. Pregnancy in women with pre-existing lupus nephritis: predictors of fetal and maternal outcome. Nephrol Dial Transplant 2009; **24**:519-25. DOI: 0.1093/ndt/gfn348

[29] Chakravarty EF, Colón I, Langen ES, et al. Factors that predict prematurity and preeclampsia in pregnancies that are complicated by systemic lupus erythematosus. Am J Obstet Gynecol 2005; **192**:1897-1904. DOI: 10.1016/j.ajog.2005.02.063

[30] Phipps E, Prasanna D, Brima W, et al. Preeclampsia: updates in pathogenesis, definitions, and guidelines. Clin J Am Soc Nephrol 2016; 11:1102-1113. DOI: 10.2215/CJN.12081115

[31] Khadijeh P, Sharareh R, Niakan K, Mahmoud A. A clinical decision support system for prediction of pregnancy outcome in pregnant women with systemic lupus erythematosus. Int J Med Inform 2017; 97L: 239-246; DOI: 10.2174/1573399815666190531100012

[32] Götestam Skorpen C, Hoeltzenbein M, Tincani A, *et al.* The EULAR points to consider for use of antirheumatic drugs before pregnancy, and during pregnancy and lactation. Ann Rheum Dis 2016; **75**:795-810. DOI: 10.1136/annrheumdis-2015-208840

Chapter 6

Normal Puerperium

Subrat Panda, Ananya Das, Arindam Mallik and Surajit Ray Baruah

Abstract

Puerperium is the time following delivery during which pregnancy-induced maternal anatomical and physiological changes return to the nonpregnant state. Puerperium period of 6 weeks can be divided into: (a) immediate – within 24 hours (b) early – up to 7 days (c) remote – up to 6 weeks. The puerperal effects are seen in all organs and particularly in reproductive organs. Infection and haemorrhage are the common postpartum complications. Post partum care is very important. Advice on exclusive breast feeding and contraception is also mandatory after every childbirth.

Keywords: puerperium, postpartum, breastfeeding, lactation, parity

1. Introduction

Puerperium is the time following delivery during which pregnancy-induced maternal anatomical and physiological changes return to the nonpregnant state. Its duration is understandably inexact, but is considered to range between 4 and 6 weeks. By popular use, however, the meaning usually includes the six subsequent weeks of delivery.

The word puerperium is derived from Latin—puer- child andparus bringing forth.

The postpartum period is associated with much tradition and superstition because the health of a new infant is very important to the survival of any family. Puerperium begins as soon as the placenta is expelled and lasts for approximately 6 weeks when the uterus regress almost to the non pregnant size.

Puerperium can be divided into:

a. immediate – within 24 hours.

b. early – up to 7 days.

c. remote – up to 6 weeks.

2. Physiology of the puerperium

2.1 Uterus

The uterus weighs approximately 1000 gm and has a volume of 5 L immediately after delivery, compared with its non pregnant weight of approximately 70 g m and 5–10 ml.

Just after delivery, the height of the uterine fundus is halfway between the pubic symphysis and the umbilicus. It happens because of the delivery of the fetus, placenta and amniotic fluid. Also there is loss of hormonal stimulation.

The height of the fundus just after delivery is 13.5 cm above the symphysis pubis. The level remains constantfor first 24 hours. After that, there is a steady decrease in height by 1.25 cm in 24 hours, resulting in uterus so that by the end of 2nd week the uterus becomes a pelvic organ. The rate of involution thereafter slows down getting back the uterus to normal size in 6 weeks. Just after delivery, due to the rapidly decreasing endometrial surface that is attached to the placenta, placenta gets sheared from the decidual layer. The average diameter of the placenta attached to the deciduas is 18 cm; which goes down to 9 cm in the immediate postpartum period.

For the first 3 days after delivery, the placental site is infiltrated with granulocytes and mononuclear cells. It is a reactionary change that extends into the endometrium and superficial myometrium as well.

By the 7th day, the regeneration of endometrial glands is evident, and they often appear atypical with irregular chromatin patterns, enlarged nuclei, pleomorphism and increased cytoplasm.

By the end ofthe first week, regeneration of the endometrial stroma is also evident, and mitotic figures are noted in gland epithelium. By postpartum day 16, the endometrium gets fully restored.

Just after birth, hemostasis is achieved by arterial smooth muscle contraction and compression of vessels by the involuting uterine muscle. In the first 8 days, vessels in the placental site are characterized by thrombosis, hyalinization. Endophlebitis in the veins and hyalinization and obliterativefibrinoid endarteritis in the arteries are notable findings.

The postpartum uterine discharge, or lochia, begins as a flow of blood that lasts several hours, then rapidly diminishes to a reddish brown discharge through the third or fourth day postpartum.

The post partum discharge is termed lochia and it contains erythrocytes, shredded decidua, epithelial cells and bacteria. For the first few days after delivery, it is known as lochia rubra. After 3 or 4 days, lochia becomes progressively pale in color and is known as lochia serosa. Then at around 10th day, because of an admixture of leukocytes and reduced fluid content, lochia assumes a white or yellow-white color known as lochia alba. The average duration of puerperial lochial discharge is from 24 to 36 days [1].

Breastfeeding or the use of oral contraceptive agents does not affect the duration of lochia. The cervical os contracts slowly, and for a few days just after labor, it readily admits two fingers. Gradually, this opening narrows and the cervix thickens with reformation of endocervical canal in a week. The external os never resumes its pre gravid appearance. It remains somewhat wider with the ectocervical depressions getting permanent at the site of lacerations.

2.2 Birth canal

The vagina and the introitus gradually reduce in size but hardly regain the nulliparous size and shape. Rugae start appearing by the third week but are less prominent. The hymen is represented by several small tissue tags of tissue that form the myrtiform caruncles.

After delivery, the vaginal epithelium reflects the hypoestrogenic state, and it stops proliferating until 4 to 6 weeks. Some damage to the pelvic floor may be inevitable, and parturition predisposes to urinary incontinence and pelvic organ prolapse.

2.3 Ovarian function

Ovulation starts as early as 27 days after childbirth. It can start after about 70 to 75 days in non lactating women. But for breastfeeding women, the mean time to ovulation can be about 6 months.

Menstruation usually resumes by 12 weeks postpartum in 70% of non lactating women. The mean time to the first menses after childbirth is 7 to 9 weeks.

In a woman exclusively breastfeeding, the likelihood of ovulation within the first 6 months postpartum is 1% to 5%.

The persistent elevation of serum prolactin in lactating women is the basis for ovulation suppression in lactating women. Prolactin levels get back to the normal range by 3 weeks after delivery in nonlactating women but remains elevated till the 6th week in lactating women.

2.4 Peritoneum and abdominal wall

The broad and round ligaments require considerable time to recover from stretching and loosening during pregnancy.

After cesarean delivery, a 6-week interval to allow fascia to heal and abdominal soreness to diminish is reasonable.

Silvery abdominal striae commonly develop as striaegravidarum.

Marked separation of the rectus abdominis muscles—diastasis recti—may result.

2.5 Blood and blood volume

Marked leukocytosis and thrombocytosis may occur during and after labor. The greatest level of coagulability is observed immediately after delivery and remains for the following 48 hours. Fibrinogen concentrations gradually diminish over the first 2 weeks postpartum. Increased fibrinolytic activity is seen in the initial 4 days following delivery. The fibrinolytic activity is back to normal in a week and is shown by plasminogen activation inhibitor 1levels. D-dimer levels are more than pregnancy levels, but are a poor marker of thrombus formation. Protein-S levels and activated protein-C resistance are less for around 6 weeks in puerperium. The changes in the coagulation system, together with vessel trauma and immobility, account for the increased risk for thromboembolism noted in the puerperium, especially when an operative delivery has occurred.

2.6 Cardiovascular system

Plasma volume is diminished by about 1000 mL just after delivery and that is due to blood loss during delivery.

Due to the shift of extracellular fluid into the vascular space. The plasma volume is replenished by the 3rd day of puerperium. Also, the total blood volume declines by 16% of the pre delivery value, and that manifests as transient anemia.

By 8 weeks of puerperium, the red cell mass rebounds and the hematocrit becomes normal in most women. Since, the blood volume becomes normal, venous tone also gets to baseline. Pulse rate increases throughout gestation, like stroke volume and cardiac output. Just after delivery, these remain elevated or may rise even higher for initial 30 to 60 minutes. Following delivery, a transient rise of about 5% occurs in both diastolic and systolic blood pressures and that continues for the first 4 days postpartum.

2.7 Thyroid function

Thyroid volume increases to about 30% during pregnancy and then gets back to normal in a 12-week period in puerperium. Both thyroxine and triiodothyronine increase throughout pregnancy and becomes normal within 4 weeks post delivery. For women on thyroid medications, it is advisable to check thyroid profile at 6 weeks postpartum to titrate the dosage. Sometimes, during the postpartum period, there is an increased risk for the development of a transient autoimmune thyroiditis that may later evolve into permanent hypothyroidism.

2.8 Immune system

The immune system gets compromised during pregnancy—particularly cellular-mediated immunity. The rebound of cellular mediated immunity after delivery leads to "flare-ups" of autoimmune diseases and subclinical infections with inflammatory reactions. Autoimmune thyroiditis, multiple sclerosis, and lupus erythematosus are examples of auto immune diseases that show flare ups in the first few months of puerperium.

2.9 Urinary tract

Normal pregnancy-induced glomerular hyperfiltration persists during the puerperium but returns to prepregnancy baseline by 2 weeks [2].

Dilated ureters and renal pelves return to their prepregnant state by 2 to 8 weeks postpartum.

Postpartum, the bladder has an increased capacity and a relative insensitivity to intravesical pressure. Thus, over distention, incomplete emptying, and excessive residual urine are frequent in puerperium [3, 4].

2.10 Lactation

Breasts begin to secrete colostrum after delivery. It is a dark yellow liquid and usually can be expressed from the nipples by the second postpartum day. In comparison to mature milk, colostrum is rich in both immunological components and minerals and amino acids [5]. It also has more protein, mostly globulin, but contains less sugar and fat.

Colostrum secretion continues for 5 days to 2 weeks post partum, with later conversion from "transitional" to mature milk in next 4 to 6 weeks.

3. Management of puerperium

3.1 Hospital stay

For most parturients, the immediate puerperium is spent in the hospital or birthing center.

In the 1950s, the lying-in period after delivery used to be around 8 to 14 days. Now, most women stay in the hospital only for 24 to 48 hours after a vaginal birth. For patients with an uncomplicated postoperative course after caesarean delivery, the post partum stay is only 2 to 4 days. During the hospital stay, the focus should be on preparation of the mother for newborn care, infant feeding including the special issues involved with breastfeeding, and also the required newborn laboratory testing.

There are no dietary restrictions for women who have been delivered vaginally. Two hours after uncomplicated vaginal delivery, a woman is allowed to eat.

3.2 Postpartum complications

Infection commonly occurs in approximately 5% of post partum patients and significant immediate postpartum hemorrhage in approximately 1% of patients. Just after the delivery of the placenta, the uterus is palpated bimanually to ascertain its tonicity. Uterine palpation is very important and is repeated frequently during the immediate postpartum period to prevent and identify uterine atony promptly. In only 1% of cases, bleeding persists or is excessive and is called delayed postpartum hemorrhage. If the bleeding is heavy or the uterus is believed to contain blood clots, uterus should be massaged until it contracts and the clots expressed. The physician may be notified, and on order an oxytocin preparation such as syntocinon 1 ml given intramuscularly orIV infusion with 5% glucose is administered. When the general condition of the mother is satisfactory, the mother and baby should be transferred to the ward. As soon as the post natal ward is notified that the newly delivered mother and her baby is to be transferred to the ward, the mid wife should arrange for a bed to be prepared in a single room or in a quite area of a ward so that the mother will be able to sleep following her efforts during delivery.

On arrival, we should note the following:

- Consistency of the uterus
- Blood loss
- Pulse
- BP
- Temperature
- General condition of the mother-tired –feeling weak
- Parity and age
- Blood group and Rh factor
- Events of labour and delivery including the amount of blood loss
- The baby's condition at birth and his birth weight
- Mother's chosen method of infant feeding
- What examinations and tests have already been carried out and plan for those which must be done during the next few days.

3.3 Daily examination

Every morning the mother should be seen and asked as to how she is feeling. The midwife should particularly note if the mother complains of feeling unduly tired. Any woman who is anaemic or who is developing an infection will not feel well. Temperature, pulse and Blood pressure should be measured. The temperature and pulse rate may be recorded at least twice a day for the few days and then once daily until the 10th days of the puerperium. If the temperature exceeds 37.3 degree Celsius or 99 degree Fahrenheit, the physician is to be notified. The pulse rate is normally 80 or below per minute. Any rise in the pulse rate above 90 beats per minute should be reported to the physician irrespective of whether it is accompanied by rise in temperature or not. Any rise in temperature may be indicative of excessive bleeding or of a developing puerperal infection. Tachycardia which is due to excessive bleeding will be accompanied by hypotension. When a nurse notices a rising pulse rate and fall in blood pressure she must check the state of the uterus and lochia in order to identify post partumhaemorrhage. The blood pressure is checked during the first 24 hours following a normal delivery and for a longer period of time, if there has been any history of bleeding, hypertension during pregnancy, or if the mother has had a Caesarean section or has required any other surgical intervention.

The breasts should be examined daily and noted whether the breasts are soft and are free from lumps, redness and soreness.

3.4 Breasts problems: sore and damaged nipples

Abnormal nipples: Inverted and flat nipples.

The complications of breast feeding are engorgement of breasts. In breasts feeding mothers breast engorgement occurs around the third and fourth post partum day. The breasts arehard, painful and sometimes flushed. The mother may develop pyrexia along with that. Engorgement results from an increased amount of blood and edema in the breasts and indicates that the baby is not ready to take the full quantity. Warm compresses to the breasts and removal of excess milk at the end of each feeding will relieve the condition. Even tight brassieres help.

3.5 The Bowels

The bowels tends to be sluggish during the puerperium for the following reasons.

1. The woman is losing fluid from her body in quantities of urine, in perspiration and breastmilk.

2. The anus maybe insensitive to stimulation having been forcibly dilated by the pressure of baby's head.

It is good to give some mild laxative for the first 36 hrs after delivery such as liquid paraffin or milk of magnesia. When diet contains sufficient roughage and fluid, the bowel needs less artificial stimulation. If the bowels do not move 48 hrs after delivery, glycerine or dulcolex suppository is usually given.

3.6 Diet

The nursing mother needs a liberal nourishing diet to build up her strength and enable her to produce sufficient breast milk. Good whole food is essential containing sufficient proteins, minerals and vitamins. As so many women are anaemic at this time the nurse must ensure that food rich in iron are included in the diet. The haemoglobin is estimated on 8th or 9th day. Iron supplements are usually prescribed for one month. As the woman is losing calcium when she breastfeeds, she should take adequate dietary calcium. Fruit and vegetables should be served at every meal.

3.7 Rest and sleep

The woman needs adequate rest, quietness and sleep because of the hypersensitive state of her nervous system. If kept awake by some discomfort such as after pains, haemorrhoids, or engorged breasts, the nurse should treat the cause before giving analgesics. The ward should be closed morning and afternoon for 1 hour. The patient is requested to relax and keep silent if they cannot sleep. The persistent insomnia in absence of pain should be viewed as a warning sign of ensuing puerperal psychosis at times.

3.8 Asepsis and antisepsis

Asepsis must be maintained, especially during the first week of puerperium. The woman is particularly vulnerable to infection at this time for the following reasons:

1. The uterus provides an ideal environment for the growth and multiplication of the micro organisms.

2. The lacerated and bruised tissues of the vulva and vagina being devitalised are unable to resist the invasion of organism.

3. The vaginal orifice is gaping and micro organisms can readily enter.

4. The woman's immunity is lowered because of depletion of energy, lack of sleep and food.

5. Blood loss may have been excessive.

The nurse must wear a mask when the vulva is exposed during the first week of puerperium.

The room and bed linen, the women skin and clothing should be clean. Adequate use of soap and water is the first requirement.

What to report to the physician.

- Temperature and pulse.
- Appetite and sleep
- Bowel and bladder movements
- Character of lochia
- Condition of sutured perineum
- Pain eg. In the breasts, abdomen, leg, head
- Any peculiarity in behaviour.

3.9 Perineal care

In puerperium, the woman is advised to maintain hygiene and clean the vulva from anterior to posterior toward the anus. A cool pack may be applied to the perineum to bring down edema and pain during the first 24 hours, especially in perineal laceration or an episiotomy.

3.10 After pains

Uterine involution manifests as several clinical findings. In primiparas, the uterus usually remains tonically contracted after delivery. Whereas in multiparas, the uterus contracts vigorously at intervals and manifests as afterpains, which are almost like labor pains. These pains are more pronounced as parity increases and worsen when the newborn lactates, because of oxytocin release. By the 3rd day post partum, afterpains decrease in intensity and become mild. In women with postpartum uterine infections, there may be severe and persistent after pains. Aspirin can be given with food in those cases.

Severe perineal, vaginal or rectal pain always warrants careful inspection and palpation. Hemorrhoidal veins are often congested at term. Thrombosis is common and may be promoted by second-stage pushing. Treatment for the condition includes topically applied anesthetics, warm soaks, and stool-softening agents.

3.11 Bowel and bladder function

Stool softeners may be prescribed, especially if the patient has had a fourth degree perineal tear or a laceration involving the rectal mucosaduring delivery.

Hemorrhoids are varicosities of the hemorrhoidal veins and are commonly found in puerperium. Surgical treatment may be considered only after 6 months postpartum to allow for natural involution. Sitz baths, stool softeners, and local medicinal preparations are useful alongwith reassurance.

She goes to the toilet after 6 hours to pass urine Periurethral edema after vaginal delivery may cause transitory urinary retention.

3.12 Retention of urine

3.12.1 Causes

1. Recumbent- posture and lack of privacy.

2. Stitches in perineum.

3. Bruises of bladder neck- bladder neck spasms.

4. Bladder atony.

3.12.2 Treatment

Women go to toilet or sit on bedpan withscreen. Hot and cold water bottles are applied on hypogastrium. Plenty of oral fluid to be given. Catherization if she cannot pass urine. Patients' urinary output should be monitored for the first 24 hours after delivery. If catheterization is required more than twice in the first 24 hours, placement of an indwelling catheter for 1 to 2 days is advisable. Prolonged catheterization needs to be avoided.

3.12.3 Pain, mood, and cognition

Mild analgesics containing codeine, aspirin, or acetaminophen, preferably in various combinations are given as frequently as every 4 hours during the first few days. It is fairly common for mother to exhibit some degree of depressed mood a few days after delivery termed postpartum blues. Post partum blues can be multi factorial. Mostly, anticipation, recognition, and reassurance works. This disorder is usually mild and self-limited to 2 to 3 days, but sometimes may last up to 10 days. Persistence or worsening of moods calls for evaluation for symptoms of major depression.

3.12.4 Ambulation

Postpartum patients should be encouraged to begin ambulation as soon as possible after delivery. Early ambulation helps avoid urinary retention and prevents puerperal venous thromboses and pulmonary embolism. Early ambulation is the key to faster recovery post delivery.

3.12.5 Breast care

Nipples are cleansed with sterile water and cotton swab before and after feeding. They are covered with sterile bra. In non lactating women, breast engorgement occurs in the initial days of puerperium and gradually reduces over this period. Painful breasts should be supported with a well-fitting brassiere. Ice packs and analgesics may also help relieve breast discomfort and pain. Women who do not wish to breastfeed should be encouraged to avoid nipple stimulation and advised to avoid continued manual expression of milk. Mastitis, or infection of the breast tissue, most often occurs in lactating women and manifests as sudden-onset fever, localized pain and swelling in the breast. Mastitis is associated with infection by micro organisms like *Staphylococcus aureus*, Group A or B streptococci, β Haemophilus species, and *Escherichia coli*.

Treatment includes continuation of breastfeeding or emptying the breast with a breast pump to avoid engorgement and also use of appropriate antibiotics.

3.12.6 Immunizations

Women who do not have antirubella antibody should be immunized during the immediate postpartum period [6]. Breastfeeding is not a contraindication for that.

If a patient has not received the tetanus-diphtheria acellular pertussis vaccine, or it has been at least 2 years since her last tetanus-diphtheria booster, she should be administered a dose before discharge from hospital.

If the woman is Rh-negative blood group, not isoimmunized and has given birth to a Rh-positive or weak-Rh-positive baby, 300 micrograms of anti-D immune globulin should be administered postpartum, ideally within 72 hours of delivery.

3.12.7 Post partum posture and exercise

In sitting posture she feeds her baby for sometime daily, she lies in her face for three weeks.

Deep breathing and simple movement of limbs are encouraged. Some simple exercises are practised when she feels it for after a few days to tone up abdominal and pelvic floor muscles as:-.

1. Deep breathing.

2. Abdominal wall is tightened on deep inspiration and breatheholding followed by its relaxation. This is done 10 times on floor with knees pulled up.

3. Pelvic floor muscles- Bent knees press on a pillow followed by relaxation for a number of times. Encourage erect walks.

4. Sexual intercourse is permitted with use of contraceptive following first post natalcheck up at sixth week.

3.13 Contraception

Postpartum care in the hospital should include discussion of contraception. Approximately 15% of non-nursing women are fertile at 6 weeks postpartum. Progestin preparations (oral norethindrone or depo-medroxyprogesterone acetate) have no effect or may slightly facilitate lactation. Women may consider initiating progesterone-only contraceptives at 6 weeks if breastfeeding exclusively or at 3 weeks if not exclusively.

Postpartum sterilization is performed at the time of cesarean delivery or after a vaginal delivery and should not extend the patient's hospital stay.

3.14 Sexual activity

Coitus may be resumed when the woman is pain free and comfortable. However, the risks of hemorrhage and infection are minimal at approximately 2 weeks post-partum. Women should be counseled, especially if breastfeeding, that coitus may initially be uncomfortable because of a dry vagina as a result of low estrogen levels. In such conditions, use of exogenous, water soluble lubrication is helpful.

3.15 Follow-up care

By discharge, women who had an uncomplicated vaginal delivery can resume most activities, including bathing, driving, and household functions. The American Academy of Pediatrics and the American College of Obstetricians and Gynecologists (2017) recommend a postpartum visit between 4 and 6 weeks. This has proven quite satisfactory to identify abnormalities beyond the immediate puerperium and to initiate contraceptive practices.

Advice on discharge for home:

- Exclusive breast feeding for 6 months
- Care of the newborn
- Total infant immunization for protection of infant from six killer diseases.
- Oral rehydration for mild diarrhoea

The discharge carries the following:

- Discharge slip- carrying details of the delivery and childbirth date.
- Instruction to mother on food, iron folic acid laxative.
- betadime cream is applied once daily on perineal wound at home for 7 days.
- She is instructed to put on sterile pad forlochial discharge and to return on sixth week for post natalcheck up.

She is also referred to infant immunization center for full immunization of infantsupto 10 months.

Post natal care:

3.16 Post natal examinations

First check up on discharge and second on sixth post partum week.

Mother: general health, pulse, BP, temperature breasts, uterine fundus is palpated per lower abdomen for normal involution.

Perineum is inspected and that of lochia.

Bladder and bowel functions are enquired.

Infant: weight, skin condition (jaundiced), eyes, condition of umbilical cord, feeding, stool, urination, any other problem are checked by referring to pediatric opd or paediatrician.

Second post natal check up on sixth week.

Mother and infant: duration of lochia, duration of first menses, sleep, bladder, bowel, perineal wound, breasts or bottle feeding.

Any problem of mother or baby is enquired.

Examination on mother: weight, BP, Pulse, anemia, breast, abdomen, perineum, pelvic organs.

Infants: weight, heart, lungs, umbilicus, Inj BCG are checked.

Advice on discharge: Food advices to mother, giving her a food chart and use of boiled water.

Rest, sleep, exercise and posture by mother.

Advice on contraceptives.

Breast feeding.

After delivery, the breasts start to secrete colostrum, which is a deep lemon yellow liquid usually by the second postpartum day. Compared with mature milk, colostrum is rich in immunological components and contains more minerals and amino acids, protein, much of which is globulin, but less sugar and fat. The colostrum content of immunoglobulin A (IgA) offers the newborn protection against enteric pathogens. Mature milk is a complex and dynamic biological fluid that consists of fat, proteins, carbohydrates, bioactive factors, minerals, vitamins, hormones and many other cellular products. The concentrations and contents of human milk change even during a single feed, but are affected by maternal diet and newborn age, health and needs.

A nursing mother usually produces 600 mL of milk daily. However, maternal gestational weight gain has little impact on the quantity or quality of milk. Milk is isotonic with plasma, and lactose alone accounts for half of the osmotic pressure. Essential amino acids in milk are derived from blood, and nonessential amino acids come from blood or synthesized in the mammary gland. Alpha-lactalbumin, beta-lactoglobulin and casein are some of the milk proteins. Fatty acids are synthesized in the breast alveoli from glucose and are secreted by an apocrine-like process. Though vitamins are found in human milk, but these are present in variable amounts. Vitamin K is virtually absent, and thus, an intramuscular dose is required to be given to the newborn [7].

Even the milk serum whey contains large amounts of interleukin-6. Human milk has a whey-to-casein ratio of 60:40 and that is considered ideal for absorption. Prolactin is also actively secreted into breast milk. Epidermal growth factor (EGF) found in milk is not destroyed by gastric proteolytic enzymes and hence may be absorbed to promote growth and maturation of newborn intestinal mucosa [8]. Lactoferrin, melatonin, oligosaccharides, and essential fatty acids are the other constituents of milk. The precise humoral and neural mechanisms involved in lactation are complex.

Progesterone, estrogen, and placental lactogen, as well as prolactin, cortisol, and insulin act in concert to stimulate the growth and development of the milk-secreting apparatus in lactating breasts [9]. With delivery, the maternal serum levels of progesterone and estrogen decline abruptly and significantly. The falling progesterone and estrogen levels remove the inhibitory influence on alpha-lactalbumin production and thus stimulates lactose synthase in milk. Progesterone withdrawal also allows prolactin to act unopposed and stimulates production of alpha-lactalbumin in milk. The intensity and duration of subsequent lactation are controlled, in large part, by the repetitive stimulus of nursing and emptying of milk from the breast. Prolactin is essential for lactation and women with extensive pituitary necrosis— Sheehan syndrome—does not lactate. Although after delivery, plasma prolactin levels drop to levels lower than during pregnancy, each act of suckling causes a rise in levels [10]. Suckling curtails the release of dopamine, also known as prolactin-inhibiting factor, from the hypothalamus. That in turn, also transiently induces prolactin secretion. Oxytocin is known to be secreted by the pituitary in pulsatile fashion. This oxytocin stimulates contraction of myoepithelial cells in the alveoli and small milk ducts and hence helps in milk expression. Milk ejection or letting down, is a reflex initiated especially by suckling, which stimulates the posterior pituitary to liberate oxytocin. The reflex may even be provoked by an infant cry and can be inhibited by maternal fright or stress.

3.17 Nursing

Human milk is known ideal food for newborns for it provides age-specific nutrients, immunological factors, and antibacterial substances to the newborn. Milk also helps in promoting cellular growth and differentiation. For both mother and infant, the benefits of breastfeeding are long-term and unique. World Health Organization (2011) recommends exclusive breastfeeding for up to 6 months.

3.18 Advantages of breastfeeding

Nutritional

Immunological

Developmental

Psychological

Social

Economical

Environmental

Optimal growth and development

Decrease risks for acute and chronic diseases

The Baby Friendly Hospital Initiative is an international program to promote exclusive breastfeeding. It is based on the World Health Organization (1989) Ten Steps to Successful Breastfeeding. World wide, almost 20,000 hospitals are designated as "baby-friendly hospitals.

Ten Steps to Successful Breastfeeding (Baby Friendly Hospital Initiative):

a. Have a written breastfeeding policy that is regularly communicated to all Health-care staff.

b. Train all staff in skills necessary to implement this policy.

c. Inform all pregnant women about the benefits and management of breastfeeding.

d. Help mothers initiate breastfeeding within an hour of birth.

e. Show mothers how to breastfeed and how to sustain lactation, even if they should be separated from their infants.

f. Feed newborns nothing but breast milk, unless medically indicated, and under no circumstances provide breast milk substitutes, feeding bottles, or pacifiers free of charge or at low cost.

g. Practice rooming-in, which allows mothers and newborns to remain together 24 hours a day.

h. Encourage breastfeeding on demand.

i. Give no artificial pacifiers to breastfeeding newborns.

j. Help start breastfeeding support groups and refer mothers to them.

3.19 Contraindications to breastfeeding

Nursing is contraindicated in some women who have intake of street drugs or alcohol abuse; have an infant with galactosemia; human immunodeficiency virus (HIV) infection; active, untreated tuberculosis; undergoing breast cancer treatment [11]. Breastfeeding has been recognized for some time as a mode of HIV transmission and is proscribed in developed countries in which adequate nutrition is otherwise available. Other viral infections do not contraindicate breastfeeding. Women with active herpes simplex virus may suckle their infants if there are no breast lesions and ifparticular care is directed to hand washing before nursing.

3.20 Other issues with lactation

With inverted and depressed nipples, nursing is very difficult. Here, lactiferous ducts open directly into a depression at the center of the areola. If the depression is not deep, milk can sometimes be expressed with the help of a breast pump. During the last few months of pregnancy, daily attempts can be madeto draw or "tease" the nipple out with the fingers.

Extra breasts—polymastia, or extra nipples—polythelia, may develop along the milk line or the former embryonic mammary ridge In some women, rests of accessory breast tissue may also be found in the mons pubis or vulva. In the general population, the incidence of accessory breast tissue ranges from 0.22 to 6 percent [12]. These accessory breasts are very small and are mistaken to be pigmented moles, lymphadenopathy or lipoma. However, polymastia has no obstetrical significance. But, occasional enlargement of these accessory breasts during pregnancy or postpartum cause patient discomfort and anxiety.

Galactocele is another complication wherein a milk duct gets obstructed by inspissated milk secretions. The amount is ordinarily limited, but an excess may form a fluctuant mass—a galactocele. Galactocoele may cause pressure symptoms and also form an abscess. It might get resolved spontaneously or might require aspiration.

Among individuals, the volume of milk secreted varies markedly. This depends on breast glandular development rather than maternal health. Rarely, there is a condition with complete lack of mammary secretion—agalactia. Again, mammary secretion might be excessive—polygalactia.

Author details

Subrat Panda*, Ananya Das, Arindam Mallik and Surajit Ray Baruah
Department of Obstetrics and Gynecology, NEIGRIHMS,
Shillong, Meghalaya, India

*Address all correspondence to: pandadrsubrat@rediffmail.com

References

[1] Fletcher S, Grotegut CA, James AH: Lochia patterns among normal women: a systematic review. J Womens Health (Larchmt) 21(12):1290, 2012.

[2] Hladunewich MA, Lafayette RA, Derby GC, et al: The dynamics of glomerular filtration in the puerperium. Am J Physiol Renal Physiol 286:F496, 2004.

[3] Buchanan J, Beckmann M: Postpartum voiding dysfunction: identifying the risk factors. Aust N Z JObstetGynaecol 54(1):41, 2014.

[4] Mulder FE, Hakvoort RA, Schoffelmeer MA, et al: Postpartum urinary retention: a systematic review of adverse effects and management. IntUrogynecol J 25(12):1605, 2014

[5] Ballard O, Morrow AL: Human milk composition: nutrients and bioactive factors. PediatrClinNorth Am 60(1):49, 2013

[6] Swamy G, Heine RP: Vaccinations for pregnant women. ObstetGynecol 125:212, 2015

[7] Wagner CL, Greer FR, American Academy of Pediatrics Section on Breastfeeding: Prevention ofrickets and vitamin D deficiency in infants, children, and adolescents. Pediatrics 122(5):1142,2008

[8] McCleary MJ: Epidermal growth factor: an important constituent of human milk. J Hum Lact7:123, 1991.

[9] Stuebe AM: Enabling women to achieve their breastfeeding goals. ObstetGynecol 123:643, 2014.

[10] Pang WW, Hartmann PE Initiation of human lactation: secretory differentiation and secretoryactivation. J Mammary Gland Biol Neoplasia 12:211, 2007.

[11] Faupel-Badger JM, Arcaro KF, Balkam JJ, et al: Postpartum remodeling, lactation, and breastcancer risk: summary of a National Cancer Institute-sponsored workshop. J Natl Cancer Inst 105(3):166, 201.

[12] Loukas M, Clarke P, Tubbs RS: Accessory breasts: a historical and current perspective. Am Surg 73(5):525, 2007.

Chapter 7

Principles of Midwifery Care during Virulent Outbreaks

Erhuvwukorotu S. Kollie

Abstract

In recent past virulent disease outbreaks have ravaged different parts of the world. The impact have been felt worldwide. During these outbreaks health workers are usually at high risk for contracting the infections. Rendering maternal antenatal, intrapartum, and postnatal care can be challenging during these outbreaks. Some of these disease that have debuted fearsome outbreaks in the recent past are described briefly in terms of their characteristics, pathology, and treatments. The struggles involved in containing one of the outbreaks are highlighted. The dilemma that ensued as a result of seeking for balance between obligation, heroic midwifery interventions, and sense of calling have been explored. Special emphasis is accorded to highlighting the experiences of midwives during the recent 2014–2015 Ebola outbreak in West Africa. Recommended principles to guide midwifery practices suitable for sustaining the safety of families needing midwifery care and health care providers rendering midwifery care are described.

Keywords: Outbreaks, Midwifery care, Virulence, Ebola virus disease, midwifery interventions, safety

1. Introduction

During disease outbreaks health care workers (HCWs) are play important role which is primary to the control of further debilitating conditions and the maintenance the overall health of the public; this condition cuts across all populations worldwide [1]. As part of the solution several studies have identified principles for training and preparing health care workers (HCWs) to equip them for the competent handling of these difficult situations. There is evidence that the education of HCWs, including midwives, which involves training and preparation activities is very important to ensure that populations experiencing disease outbreak survive the event and recover meaningfully to optimum community health conditions. This involve equipping HCWs with skills vital for the conduction of competent surveillance, communication, reporting, and containment of outbreaks [2, 3]. It should be noted here that midwives operate under the domain of normal pregnancies, childbirth, and peuperium however, their clinical interventions during a virulent outbreak can become complicated with the high risk for contracting deadly diseases or transmitting the diseases to their patients. Several factors influence the availability and positive response of HCWs including midwives to contribute to the containment of the disease during disease outbreaks. Some of these factors include their willingness in spite of the risks involved such as uncertainty and insecurity. Other factors are their perceptions and attitudes towards their roles during disease outbreaks [1, 4]. Scholars have identified that HCWs were somewhat willing to render care to victims during influenza virus epidemics [5–7]. Other studies have indicated differences in the rate of willingness of health workers to care for patients who are victims of virulent and life threatening epidemics, pandemics, and infectious diseases [8]. The study in [7] provided descriptions of the determinants of HCWs higher willingness to render care during epidemics; These include the type of disease outbreak (for example; it was shown that less virulent outbreaks were related with higher willingness of HCWs to continue to care for patients), also shown by studies that lower threat perceptions of health care workers are related with higher efficacy assertion (meaning higher assertion to being competent to handle the situation). It can be summarized then, that when disease outbreaks are less virulent, the threat perception of the outbreak are lower, while the self-determined ability to handle the situation becomes higher among HCWs. This results in a higher level of willingness by health care workers to continue to care for patients in the event of disease outbreaks. When outbreak of diseases were at its peak, the health care workers in close contact with victims, thereby putting them in a frontline position to salvage the situation, where recorded to express high rate of unwillingness to respond [1, 7]. One of such deadly disease outbreaks that have hit the world in recent past is the Ebola Virus disease that occurred in West Africa from 2014 to 2015. Studies to understand and describing the experiences of nurses and midwives and their willingness to care for patients during the Ebola disease outbreak have identified those factors that influenced midwives to care for patients during the fearsome outbreak [9]. It is important to note that during the Ebola outbreak in Liberia and West Africa as a whole, there was the great need to care for patients who had contracted the Ebola virus, but there was need also to pay attention to other patient populations who needed other health care services. Pregnant women, women in labor for child birth, and women who had just delivered their babies, newborn babies, and children with diverse conditions not related to Ebola were constantly in need of health care services [8].

Coping with the new disease with a recorded high mortality rate within the region, including development of treatment protocols, was a serious concern in the region. The situation was complicated further because the needed resources were not available in countries in the region (one of which was Liberia). These resource constraints included experienced experts in treatment and care for patients with Ebola. This inadequacy was caused by conditions created by the emergence from civil war in which lead to limited availability of health resources and a dysfunctional health care system in [8]. In addition, Ebola virus disease symptoms are not easily differentiated from other endemic diseases like malaria, gastroenteritis, or cholera [10]. The Ebola virus disease manifest symptoms that could be similar to other infectious diseases, meanwhile these symptoms are fatal. This caused high tension and anxiety among the health care workers and their attitude towards every patient who sought care changed in such a way that all patients were treated as suspected cases [11]. In appreciating the complexity of the new epidemic, in a statement about the Ebola outbreak in Liberia made by the World Health Organization (WHO) [12] it was reported that the highest number of deaths ocured in Liberia. This was also recorded as the most devastating outbreak of Ebola since it first emerged in 1976 in the Democratic Republic of Congo. When the epidemic reached its peak between August and September 2014, it was estimated that 300 to 400 new cases every week were reported. The situation in the country was very tragic; the treatment centers were overflowing with patients (which included women in labour, some of which delivered their babies in front of health care facilities). Horrific scenes were recorded were patients died on the hospital premises unattended to and bodies abandoned there for days. Local and International flights were cancelled, and domestic supplies of food, gas, fuel ran low. Public places such as schools, businesses offices, border control, open markets, and most health institutions were closed down. Fear and uncertainty about the future—for families, for communities, and for the country and its economy was the common feeling in the country. The health care workers continued to play their roles in the management of patients, though supplies of personal protective equipment, training and preparation for safety procedures were inadequate. This led to the report of 375 health care workers who became infected and loss of the lives of 189 HCWs [12].

The enigma of the Ebola outbreak was associated to the challenges that were then posed to HCWs within the West African Region by the International Council of Nurses (ICN) [13]. Ebola infections according to the ICN [13] were contracted by health care workers which resulted in the debilitating effects on the health system; that included the closing down of hospitals, the reduction in the health care workforce, and a distrusted health system. It was reported also that health care workers were 21–32 times more likely to be infected with Ebola than were other adults in the general population [13]. In the three countries that were affected; Liberia, Guinea, and Serra Leone, 50% of all health care workers infected were nurses, 12% were physicians and medical students, and 7% were laboratory workers. These numbers of deaths of health care workers reflected the need to improve and strengthen safety policies, supply of adequate protective equipment, and the appropriate preparation and training for all HCWs. The International Council of Nurses recommended to governments to ensure the creation of safe working environments for health care workers as a prerequisite to providing care to Ebola patients. The ICN also recommended that nurses and midwives require proper training and education, prompt provision of protective equipment, and to take up an active, frontline role in the development of policies pertaining to the prevention of infection transmission and patient care [13].

The understanding of the high risks associated with giving care to infected patients during virulent outbreaks for midwives, attention should be increased and placed on the safety issues, social processes, and the needed to develop a more realistic policy that will meet the needs of midwives. There is also the need to describe what midwives went through during the epidemic while caring for Ebola and non-Ebola patients, which involved midwives' decision making about rendering or not rendering care to patients during the Ebola outbreak. This will serve as eye opener for other midwives to appreciate and understand the principles that they would need to internalize and utilize whenever necessary to render care to women and their families who in need of midwifery care during virulent outbreaks.

2. Disease that have caused virulent outbreaks in recent past

Some of the disease that have debuted fearsome outbreaks in the recent past are described very briefly in terms of their characteristics, pathology, and treatments. These diseases include Ebola virus disease, Avian influenza, Cholera, Yellow fever, Middle East Respiratory Syndrome Coronavirus, Marburg virus disease, and Zika virus infection. The COVID-19 disease debuted in 2019 and is currently ravaging the world (**Table 1**).

2.1 Ebola virus disease

According to WHO [10] Ebola viral disease (EVD) can cause fatal complications among humans up to about 90%. Wild animals transmit the virus to humans and then human to human transmission occurs through physical interactions between

Disease outbreak	Country	Year
COVID-19	220 Countries globally	2019
Ebola Virus	Uganda, Serra Leone, Liberia, Guinea, Nigeria	2010; 2014
Avian Influenza	Egypt, Indonesia, China	2010; 2011; 2013
Cholera	Haiti, Democratic Republic of Congo	2010; 2015
Yellow Fever	Senegal, Nigeria	2011; 2017
Middle East Respiratory Syndrome Coronavirus	Middle Eastern Countries; US, Saudi	2013; 2017
Marburg Virus Disease	Uganda	2014
Zika Virus infection	Panama, Honduras, Cape Verde, Paraguay, Mexico, Guatamala	2015

Table 1.
Disease outbreaks occurrence in the past ten years.

them. The clinical manifestations of Ebola infection starts to show between 2 to 10 days after a humans contract the virus. People can only transmit the virus during the period that they are. Survival critically depends on the provision of early supportive care which include rehydration and symptomatic treatment because there is currently no standard pharmacologic treatment to destroy the virus [10]. Ebola virus disease or EVD occurred first in 1976 in two concurrent outbreaks in Eastern Africa: one in Nzara, Sudan, and the other in Yambuku, Democratic Republic of Congo [10]. EVD is caused by a virus called Filoviridae, one of the viruses included in the family of hemorrhagic fever viruses that cause uncontrolled bleeding complications accompanied with fevers. The natural host for the Ebola virus are fruit bats [14]. When humans come in close contact with the fluids such as blood, body secretions, other bodily fluids of animals such as chimpanzees, gorillas, fruit bats, monkeys, forest antelope, and porcupines that are infected by the Ebola virus and/or are found ill or dead or in the rain forest, the humans contract the virus [14]. Transmission of Ebola virus among humans occurs when humans come in direct contact with fluiids and body parts of other humans. For example when broken skin or mucous membranes of one human come into contact with the blood, secretions, or body fluids of other ihumans who are infected by the virus, even when they come in contact with materials (such as, bed clothing) contaminated with body fluids of other infected people. Once a person is infected with the virus they remain infectious throughout, as long as they virus remains in them and after death occurs due to the disease [10]. People infected with the Ebola Virus are not infectious until the symptoms begin to show, these symptoms begin to manifest between 2 to 21 days after infection. The Symptoms include headaches, fever that occurs suddenly, sore throat, muscle pain, fatigue, vomiting and diarrhea, skin rashes, clinical signs of renal and hepatic dysfunction, and internal and external bleeding (Symptoms of Ebola virus disease, para.1) [10]. The diagnosis of EVD can be difficult due to the indistinct clinical signs and symptoms compared to other infectious diseases however, laboratory tests can be used to confirm that a person in infected with the Ebola Virus. Examples of the laboratory tests that can be used to confirm EVD include antibody-capture enzyme-linked immunosorbent assay, antigen-capture detection tests, serum neutralization test, reverse transcriptase polymerase chain reaction assay, electron microscopy, and virus isolation by cell culture. EVD has no developed treatment yet. However, there is a range of potential treatments including blood products administration, immune therapies, drug therapies, and vaccines which are currently being developed. Survival depends the provision of early supportive care which include rehydration and symptomatic treatment because there is currently no standard pharmacologic treatment to destroy the virus [10]. The skills and protocols involved in nursing care for patients with EVD are undergoing development. Some scholars have suggest the following as nursing interventions emanating from the experiences of nurses who were directly involved in the care of EVD patients:

The improvements made in the treatment techniques makes it now possible to render adequate care for EVD challenged patients with much better clinical results.

1. The safety and protection of health care providers is essential therefore, there should be adequate and timely provision of personal protective gear and equipment.

2. The management of patients with EVD is multifaceted and entails the utilization of isolation technique and the use of full protective gear. This require intensive training and practice.

3. There is need to engage in elaborated communication to everyone in and around the treatment facilities which involves detailed and repeated communications. This will distill the fear related to, and the inaccuracies and exaggerated reports by media on matters concerning personal and community risk.

4. The response to the crisis created by Ebola outbreak require the encouragement of volunteerism among nurses and midwives [15].

Midwifery interventions require touch; which is the main medium that people connect with each other. Touch is an important part of the midwife-patient relationship and may be the unavoidable aspects of the caring relationship between midwives and their patients [16]. Nurses and midwives use touch to promote healing and provide comfort and care to their patients. Touching patients is done in different kind of ways during every interaction; for instance, when measuring vital signs, bathing their patients, changing positions of patients in bed, assisting patients to leave their bed to walk or sit in a chair [16]. When midwives touch their patients, especially during the Ebola outbreak, it speaks volumes in terms of reassures them that the midwife is not afraid to be near them and that they are not alone. Though direct skin-to-skin contact is not wise nor acceptable, it is recommended that when midwives treat EVD patients, despite the layers of protective equipment, they need to seek for avenues to intentionally touch their patients in a deliberate and meaningful way that will provide care, comfort and connection between the midwife and the patient [16].

Curriculum development is crucial and important so that student midwives would be given a robust understanding of the knowledge, skills, and attitudes necessary to care for patients in the event of public health emergencies like the Ebola outbreak. For instance, Teachers at Emory's Nell Hodgson Woodruff School of Nursing worked is collaboration with their colleagues at the Centers for Disease Control and Prevention (CDC) to create and deliver a course that they titled, "Introduction to Complex Humanitarian Emergencies for Nurses." This course utilized presentations and active learning exercises that examined the methods needed to provide and manage public health emergency situations that require prompt care and opportunities for leadership. This could be applied and contextualized to midwifery and nursing schools in West Africa and globally as a continuous education program to update and improve midwifery care during disease outbreaks [17].

2.2 Avian influenza

The avian influenza viruses are zoonotic influenza viruses are resident in birds and cause Avian influenza commonly called bird flu. These animal influenza viruses are distinct from human seasonal influenza viruses and they do not easily become contagious and transmit from human to human. Occasionally through direct or indirect contact they infect humans and cause diseases that could lead to death. Avian influenza A(H5N1) first outbreak was in 1997 in a poultry in Hong Kong. It became widespread in 2003 from Asia to Europe to Africa. A(H5N1) occurs naturally in wild waterfowl, but it can spread easily to domestic poultry. The disease is transmitted to humans through contact with infected bird feces, nasal secretions, or secretions from the mouth or eyes. Also it is suspected that bird flu could be contacted by consuming improperly cooked poultry or eggs from infected birds, eggs should never be served runny. Bird meat when not properly cooked to an internal temperature of 165°F (73.9°C) could pose a risk. Symptoms of bird flu include cough, diarrhea, respiratory difficulties, fever (over 100.4°F or 38°C), headache, muscle aches, malaise, runny nose, and sore throat. Treatments may vary because different types of avian influenza can cause different symptoms. Most times antiviral medication such as oseltamivir (Tamiflu) or zanamivir (Relenza) can help alleviate the severity of the disease, especially when the medication is taken within 48 hours after symptoms first appear. Further management would be to place those infected in isolation to avoid spreading the virus to others [18].

2.3 Cholera

Cholera is an acute form of diarrhoeal disease, if not treated it can kill within hours. Several studies have identified approximately that every year there are 1.3 million to 4.0 million cases of cholera, and 21 000 to 143 000 deaths worldwide due to cholera. Most cases presents no or mild symptoms. Treatment with oral rehydration solution would be effective in such cases. More severe cases will require quick and immediate treatment with intravenous fluids and antibiotics. Control measures involve the provision of safe water and sanitation, safe oral cholera vaccines, improvements in water and sanitation [19].

2.4 Yellow fever

Yellow fever is caused by a virus found in parts of Africa and South America. The virus is spread to people by the bite of a mosquito. Symptoms of the illness ranges from fever with aches and pains to severe liver disease with bleeding and yellow colored skin (known as jaundice). Yellow fever presents first set of symptoms which include sudden onset of fever, chills, severe headache, back pain, general body aches, nausea, vomiting, fatigue, and weakness. Most persons improve after the initial presentation. After a brief remission ranging from hours to a day, about 15% of infection cases progress to develop sever symptoms which include high fever, jaundice, bleeding, and eventually shock and failure of multiple organs. Treatment is symptomatic and includes provision of rest, fluids, and use of pain relievers and medication to reduce fever to relieve symptoms of aching and fever. Yellow fever patients should be hospitalized for supportive care and close observation, they should be provided with material to protect them from more mosquito bites (by encouraging that they stay indoors and stay under a mosquito net). This should be adhered to for up to 5 days after the symptoms like fever begins. This will allow the yellow fever virus in their bloodstream to be unavailable to uninfected mosquitoes, thereby putting a halt to the further transmission of the virus and containing the risks posed to other people around the patients. There is no medicine to treat the infection yet. Prevention is advisory which include use insect repellent, wear long-sleeved shirts and long pants outdoors, and get vaccinated. The incubation period (time from infection until illness) when people get infected is typically 3–6 days [20].

2.5 Middle East Respiratory Syndrome Coronavirus

This is a respiratory disease caused by a group of viruses known as coronaviruses discovered first in the Middle East region, specifically Saudi Arabia in 2012. These coronaviruses constitute a large family of viruses that can cause different kinds of diseases such as the common cold and Severe Acute Respiratory Syndrome (SARS). The clinical manifestations of Middle East Respiratory Syndrome Coronavirus (MERS-CoV) include cough, fever, and shortness of breath. Other symptoms include pneumonia, and some gastrointestinal complications such as diarrhea. There are cases when infected people go on asymptomatic, meaning that they do not present any clinical signs nor symptoms, but they test positive for MERS-CoV after a laboratory test is conducted. In order to track down these asymptomatic cases rigorous contact tracing of a laboratory-confirmed case should be done. It is reported that so far about 35% of confirmed MERS-CoV infected patients have died. Transmission is mainly through human-to-human infections especially in health care settings; when providing unprotected care to a patient. Health care associated outbreaks have debuted in several countries, with the largest outbreaks seen in Saudi Arabia, United Arab Emirates, and the Republic of Korea. Scientific evidence have suggested that dromedary camels are a major reservoir host for MERS-CoV and have transmitted MERS infection to humans [21].

2.6 Marburg virus disease

Marburg virus disease (MVD) was formerly known as Marburg hemorrhagic fever. This is a severe fatal illness in humans transmitted to humans by *Rousettus aegyptiacus*, a fruit bat of the Pteropodidae family. It spreads among humans through human-to-human transmission. The average MVD case fatality rate is recored at around 50%. Community engagement is critical to successfully controlling outbreaks. To achieve good outbreak control several sets of interventions should be considered which include case management, infection prevention and control practices, surveillance and contact tracing, a good laboratory service, safe burials, and social mobilization. Early supportive care with rehydration, symptomatic treatment improves survival. No treatment has yet been developed [22].

2.7 Zika virus infection

Zika virus infectious disease is caused by a virus transmitted mainly by *Aedes* mosquitoes. Infected people present symptoms which include mild fever, skin rash, conjunctivitis, muscle and joint pain, malaise or headache. The symptoms usually last for 2–7 days. Zika can be transmitted from a pregnant woman to her fetus. Infection during pregnancy can cause certain birth defects such as microcephaly and Guillain-Barré syndrome. There is no vaccine or medicine for Zika virus infection [23, 24].

2.8 COVID-19 Disease

COVID-19 disease also known as Coronavirus disease is an infectious disease caused by a newly discovered virus called coronavirus. It is spread by droplet transmission from one human to another who are in close physical interaction. The COVID-19 virus is spread primarily through droplets of saliva or discharge from the nose when an infected person coughs or sneezes. It's important that people practice respiratory etiquette (for example, by coughing into a flexed elbow). People who get infected with the COVID-19 virus experience mild to moderate respiratory illness and recover without requiring special treatment. Special populations of humans are affected differently; ie older people, and those with underlying medical problems like diabetes, chronic respiratory disease, cardiovascular disease, and cancer are more likely to develop serious physiological responses. Prevention of transmission is best achieved by slowing down transmission by ensuring that the population is informed about the COVID-19 virus, the disease it causes and how it spreads. Other protective measures include washing hands or using an alcohol based rub frequently using facial mask, and not touching the face. The most common symptoms include fever, dry cough, tiredness. There are less common symptoms such as aches and pains, sore throat, diarrhoea, conjunctivitis, headache, loss of taste or smell and a rash on skin, or discoloration of fingers or toes. More serious symptoms also showcase such; difficulty breathing or shortness of breath, chest pain or pressure, loss of speech or movement. It takes an average of 5–6 days from when an individual is infected with the virus for symptoms to show, however it can take up to 14 days. Treatment mostly is by symptoms An approved drug, remdesivir (Veklury) is used to treat COVID-19. Any treatments that are used for COVID-19 should be taken under the care of a healthcare provider [25].

3. The experiences of midwives during a disease outbreak

Before elaborating on the principles that will guide midwifery care during virulent outbreaks. Let us appreciate the experiences of midwives during the 2-14-2015 Ebola virus disease outbreak in Liberia, West Africa. It is from this backdrop that the principles of midwifery care during virulent outbreaks are proposed. A study described the experiences of midwives during the EVD outbreak in Liberia; the midwives were living and working in fear and terror; their lives and those of their families were endangered [9]. The key concern of the midwives were concern for their family's safety, psychological, emotional, and social support. The midwives mostly felt obligated by virtue of their profession to continue caring for patients during the Ebola outbreak [9]. The midwives experienced stigmatization by the public during the outbreak due to fear of many that the midwives stood a greater risk to transmit the disease to their families and the public in general. However after engaging in the education of their families and patients, together with institutional influences, and government efforts eased the effect of stigmatization [9]. There is need for governments to improve their efforts to develop policies, provide safe working conditions, and fund training and educational programs in Ebola care [26].

Midwives experienced changes in the dynamics of the midwife-patient relationship and working in teams during the period of the outbreak. The training and education of the midwives, also the provision of protective equipment assisted the midwives to regain their confidence and self-efficacy. The midwives found ways to touch all patients despite the high risk involved, while using the personal protective equipment provided. They conducted midwifery procedures fully, improved the relationship between themselves and their patients. The spiritual dimension of health care was identified in a study as crucial to enhancing midwives' well-being [9]. Other authors have also reported that faith-based health care institutions and services are the vehicle used to drive spiritual health care [27]. The decision process involved in the midwives' choices either to render care or not to render care for patients were made on the basis of emotional connections between them and other midwives and nurses, their families, and society. The decision process also was based on their value system, including professionalism and spirituality. The findings of the Kollie, Winslow, Porthier, and Geade study indicated the spiritual resources of midwives had influence on their decision to work. The study identified a conceptual map which described the work decision process to include that the midwives were in a state of fear and terror. Their situation was associated with emotional and psychological dimensions of the fear and terror condition [9]. Several factors were shown to influence their decision to work; key among them the family. Midwives made decisions to either work or not during the Ebola outbreak based on family responsibilities and demands. The midwives decided to work as a result of their sense of professionalism and their realization that the needed to depend on God for safety. There were institutional influences and also government roles which was shown to have both positive and negative influences on whether the midwives decided to work or not. The midwives decision to work was influenced by stigmatization issues which caused sadness and frustration. Stigmatization however did not stand out as a reason for the midwives to decide to stop working during the Ebola outbreak. Those midwives who continued to work during the outbreak encountered changes in the relationship between the patients and themselves as well as, midwives. Further description of the factors that influenced the midwives to continue to render care to their patients during the fearsome and dreadful 2014–2015 Ebola virus disease outbreak [9] are as follows:

3.1 Living in fear and terror

The midwives felt afraid and terrorized by the possibility of contracting the disease through interaction with patients and colleagues, and transmitting it to family members.

3.2 Family

The fear for their family's safety made the situation difficult for the midwives. In order to alleviate their fears and prevent the possible transmission of the virus to their family members, midwives bathed upon their return home and before they began to interact with members of their family. This phenomenon created what was described as physical distancing between their spouses and children, this was very difficult for them to endure, especially when they considered great risk the situation posed to their family. The results of the study identified that the midwives considered the physical distancing as the responsible thing to do; to ensure their family's safety irrespective of their desire for affection and closeness from their family members. The primary reason for a midwife to stop working during the outbreak was identified as family. The discouragement from family members or the sense of family responsibility was identified as the key factor that influenced those who did not work or stopped after a period of working.

3.3 Professionalism

The midwives were passionate for their profession, love for people, and sympathy or empathy for sick people. Financial benefits were not the motivation. The Midwives' logic for continuing to work was that their refusal to work would eventually lead to genocide, that neither they nor their relatives would be spared; that would be the retribution. The situation provided the opportunity for the midwife to gain additional clinical experience, competence, and confidence.

3.4 God and safety

The midwives depended on God for safety. This was the primary resource for safety, despite the availability of protective equipment. They believed that the surety of protection was only possible through dependence on God.

3.5 Stigmatization

People in society realized that the midwives were at risk of contracting infection and could in turn spread the virus to the public. This led to the stigmatization of the midwives and resulted in feelings of fear, frustration, and sadness.

3.6 Institutional influences

When hospitals closed because of fear, unpreparedness, and possible high risk of transmission to staff, the midwives felt the opportunity to continue serving was closed.

3.7 Government efforts

The government came through with their responsibility to provide Personal protective equipment. The government failed to deliver on its promise to compensate the workers with hazard allowance.

4. Principles that guide midwifery care during virulent outbreaks

The principles that guide midwifery care during virulent outbreaks will be discussed generally for all virulent disease outbreaks. These general principles will offer basic safety and educational guidelines that cut across all virulent outbreaks. During virulent outbreaks health workers are usually at high risk for contracting the infections. This poses a great risk to their patients, family members, and themselves. Rendering maternal antenatal, intrapartum, and postnatal care and immediate newborn care would be challenging during these outbreaks. The struggles involved in containing the outbreaks involves the dilemma of seeking for balance between obligation, heroic midwifery interventions, and the sense of professional calling. The solution would be to guide midwifery practice with fundamental principles to serve as frameworks for contextual evidence based midwifery interventions during deadly disease outbreaks.

These principles are discussed under domains of midwifery care; antenatal, intrapartum, postnatal, and immediate newborn care. General safety and education issues will also be explained.

4.1 Antenatal care

The care for pregnant women and their growing fetus is needful to ensure the desired outcome of a healthy pregnancy and fetus. The management of pregnancy during antenatal care during virulent outbreaks should be guided by the following principles:

1. Initial mandatory sensitivity screening test for all virulent infections such as Cholera, COVID-19, Ebola virus infection, and so on should conducted to rule

out cases of infective patients. This involves the history taking and temperature screening for all women.

2. Health education should no longer be conducted in physical group classes, the option of virtual group classes, or sharing of screen casts of health education classes could be explored. This is because more recent virulent outbreaks have been of diseases that are easily transmitted via air and fluid droplets (COVID-19 and Ebola). Moreover, the transmission of such recent outbreaks have been aided by interpersonal physical contact. Social distancing has been prescribed by the WHO recently [25]. Individual appointments for educational activities should be conducted. Where the condition permits educational activities could adopt other forms including phone conversations, use of the internet through the hospital website or email services to the clients, and distribution of video clips on salient health topics to mothers.

3. Physical assessment procedures such as general head-to-toe examination, abdominal examination, and laboratory tests should be conducted under strict protective conditions. The use of the basic personal protective gears, and continuous sterilization of the examination rooms should be practiced. Blood and body fluid samples should be handled with great care.

4. The examination of fetal wellbeing should be conducted under protective conditions.

4.2 Intrapartum (delivery) care

As soon as labour is established, the woman is advised to report to the hospital. The midwife is responsible to assess, plan, and implement care to address physical, emotional, and support needs of the woman in labour. In the first stage of labour the assessment procedures should include history taking, general examination, abdominal examination, vaginal examination, and fetal assessment. At admission history is taken first on behavioral patterns that might have put the mother at risk of contracting a virulent infection. Other history on details from previous births and babies, characteristics of uterine contractions (frequency, duration, and perception of strength), ruptured membrane/color and amount of amniotic fluid, vaginal discharge, fetal movement, medical history can follow.

Support from the relatives of the woman in labor should be encouraged so as to boost the woman's confidence and help her in decision making. However it is advised that all relatives stay out of the delivery room to reduce the risk of transmitting diseases or infections.

Procedures should be conducted under a clean field. Personal protective gears should be worn by the midwife always. All materials used should be clean. Mother can be encouraged to take a bath and clean the perineal area. Mothers and relatives should be required to wear protective masks at all times. This is predicated on the novel COVID-19 infections. Regular hand-washing and hand- sanitization should be ensured for mothers and relatives to prevent transmission of all types of diseases and virulent infections.

Vaginal examination should be conducted under aseptic measures. A full explanation of the procedure is given to the woman and her consent obtained. Take note of discharges or bleeding from the vaginal orifice, note the amount, excessive amount may indicate suspicion of symptoms of hemorrhagic fevers (EVD).

In the second stage of labor as long as the mother and baby are well, and there is good progress in labour, then the outcome will be good. The management of the second stage of labour consist of positioning, delivery of the head, and delivery of the shoulders and the rest of the body.

The management of the third stage of labour involves two main protocols: the use of uterotonics for the prevention of postpartum hemorrhage (PPH) during the third stage of labour is recommended for all births. Oxytocin (10 IU, IV/IM) is the recommended uterotonic drug for the prevention of PPH. In the situation where excessive bleeding does not respond to interventions and other physiologic indicators for bleeding are ruled out, caution should be applied to suspected EVD symptoms.

The second protocol is controlled cord traction (CCT) is recommended for vaginal births to achieve a small reduction in blood loss and a small reduction in the duration of the third stage of labour.

4.3 Postnatal care

The continuous screening and preventive measures for virulent diseases and infections continues in addition to typical postnatal care protocols; postnatal visitation appointment, infant feeding, reproductive and contraceptive plan, pregnancy complications follow-up care, postpartum complications detection and management, and mental health care. During postnatal care visitations the following should be observed by the midwives, mothers, and their relatives to prevent transmission of virulent infections; regular hand-washing or hand-sanitization, temperature checks, use of protective nose masks, social distancing, and barrier midwifery care (which involves the use of gloves, googles, boots, and masks).

4.4 Immediate newborn care

This could be summarized to include wiping, drying, warming (ideally skin-to-skin contact) and wrapping. Providing skin-to-skin contact is indicated only for mothers and babies who test negative to any virulent infection. Evaluating breathing and resuscitation if necessary as usual in the management of the newborn infant. Use a sterile method to cut the cord and evaluate bleeding from the cord area as suggestive of possible EVD symptoms. The management of the newborn infant also include initiating exclusive breastfeeding in the first hour for infants whose mothers have been confirmed negative to virulent infection screening.

4.5 General safety and education

The safety and education of midwives, health care workers, mothers and their relatives should be assured by conducting several general safety and education activities. Some of these activites include;

- initial screening for all virulent infections to serve as baseline data for all health care workers and midwifery clients of the health care facility

- daily temperature screening for all health care workers and midwifery clients of the health care facility

- compulsory regular hand-washing or hand-sanitization for all health workers and midwifery clients (immediately after every activity in the health care facility)

- use of nose mask by all midwifery clients at all times in the health care facility
- use of protective gears such as googles, nose masks, gloves, boots, at all times in the health care facility
- use of basic personal protective gears by all midwives and health care workers during procedures
- Posting of easy-to-read information posters about all virulent diseases that have caused outbreaks recently in all spaces and locations within the health care facility
- Preparation and distribution of educational materials about virulent infections and diseases such as screen casts, fliers, SMS to all registered midwifery clients of the health care facility

The unique clinical skills which emerged from the perspective of the midwives working during the Ebola outbreak in Liberia [9] could be incorporated in the training of students midwives. This includes the training of hand washing techniques, and wearing and use of both basic and enhanced personal protective gears. There is need for nursing and midwifery professional boards and regulatory bodies to continue to assure continuous education on virulent infections preventive care and safety measures for midwives. Curricula in the schools of midwifery should include preventive care and safety measures. This could involve the training on the management of midwife-patient relationships, empowering midwife-midwife relationships, the proper use of the both basic and enhanced personal protective equipment and protective measures, and adjustment techniques. The training for virulent infections preventive care and safety measures should also involve ethical considerations and mental or psychological indications. Community health education on recent virulent disease outbreaks could be conducted by midwives to help communities understand the diseases and improve behavior towards health care workers. The role that faith plays in the decisions made by midwives should also be recognized when developing and implementing curricula.

5. Conclusion

Virulent disease outbreaks result in dreadful risks for contracting contagious diseases or infections to health workers including midwives. This poses a great risk to their patients, family members, and themselves. The struggles involved in containing the outbreaks involves the dilemma of seeking for balance between obligation, heroic midwifery interventions, and the sense of professional calling. Rendering maternal antenatal, intrapartum, and postnatal care and immediate newborn care would be challenging during these outbreaks. The solution would be to guide midwifery practice with fundamental principles to serve as frameworks for contextual evidence based midwifery interventions during deadly disease outbreaks.

Conflict of interest

The author declares on conflict of interest.

Author details

Erhuvwukorotu S. Kollie
Adventist University of West Africa, Schiefflin Township, Margibi, Liberia

*Address all correspondence to: kolliee@auwa.edu.lr

References

[1] Barnett, D. J., Thompson, C. B., Errett, N. A., Semon, N. L., Anderson, M. K., Ferrell, J. L., ... Links, J. M: Determinants of emergency response willingness in the local public health workforce by jurisdictional and scenario patterns; A cross-sectional survey. BMC Public Health. 2012;12, 164. Doi: 10.1186/1471-2458-12-164

[2] Chiu, M., Polivka, B.J., & Stanley S.A.R: Evaluation of a disaster: Surge training for public health nurses. Public Health Nursing. 2011;29 (2), 136-142.

[3] Qureshi, K. A., Gershon, R. R., Yamada, S., & Li, D: Factors related to essential workers' ability and willingness to work and comply with personal infection control protocol during a large scale influenza pandemic in Hawaii. Journal of Emergency & Disaster Medicine. 2013; 2, 1.

[4] Devnani, M: Factors associated with the willingness of health care personnel to work during an influenza public health emergency: An integrative review. Prehospital Disaster Medicine. 2012;27(6), 551-566. Doi: 10.1017/s1049023x12001331

[5] Balicer, R. D., Barnett, D. J., Thompson, C. B., Hsu, E. B., Catlett, C. L., Watson, C. M., ... Links, J. M: Characterizing hospital workers' willingness to report to duty in an influenza pandemic through threat- and efficacy-based assessment. BMC Public Health. 2010;10, 436. Doi: 10.1186/1471-2458-10-436

[6] Barnett, D. J., Balicer, R. D., Thompson, C. B., Storey, J. D., Omer, S. B., Semon, N. L., ... Links, J. M: Assessment of local public health workers' willingness to respond to pandemic influenza through application of the extended parallel process model. PLoS One. 2009;4(7), e6365. Doi: 10.1371/journal.pone.0006365

[7] Basta, N. E., Edwards, S. E., & Schulte, J: Assessing public health department employees' willingness to report to work during an influenza pandemic. Journal of Public Health Management Practice. 2009;15(5), 375-383. Doi: 10.1097/PHH.0b013e3181a391e2

[8] Buseh, A. G., Stevens, P. E., Bromberg, M., & Kelber, S. T: The Ebola epidemic in West Africa: Challenges, opportunities, and policy priority areas. Nursing Outlook. 2015;63(1), 30-40. Doi: 10.1016/j.outlook.2014.12.013

[9] Kollie, E.S., Winslow, B.J., Pothier, P. & Gaede, D: Deciding to work during the Ebola outbreak: The voices and experiences of nurses and midwives in Liberia. International Journal of Africa Nursing Sciences. 2017. DOI:10.1016/j.ijans.2017.09.002

[10] World Health Organization factsheet. Ebola Virus Disease. n.d. Available from: http://www.who.int/mediacentre/factsheets/fs103/en/[Accessed: 2015-08-11]

[11] Hayter, M: Ebola—The best and the worst within nursing ... and maybe us all. Nursing Outlook. 2015; *63*(1), 8-9. Doi: 10.1016/j.outlook.2014.11.009

[12] World Health Organization statement. The Ebola outbreak in Liberia is over. 2015. Available from: http://www.who.int/mediacentre/news/statements/2015/liberia-ends-ebola/en/[Accessed: 2015-05-9]

[13] International Council of Nurses. Ebola: Protect our nurses! International Council of Nurses calls for greater support for frontline healthcare workers. 2015. Available from: http://www.icn.ch/images/stories/documents/

news/press_releases/2015_PR_11_Ebola_WHO_report.pdf [Accessed: 2015-05-9]

[14] Borio, L., Inglesby, T., Peters, C.J., Schmaljohn, A.L., Hughes, J.M., Jahrling, P.B., ...Tonat, K: Hemorrhagic fever viruses as biological weapons- Medical and public health management. Journal of American Medical Association. 2002;287(18), 2391-2405.

[15] Matlock, A. M., Gutierrez, D., Wallen, G., & Hastings, C: Providing nursing care to Ebola patients on the national stage: The National Institutes of Health experience. Nursing Outlook. 2015;63(1), 21-24. Doi: 10.1016/j.outlook.2014.11.015

[16] Connor, A: Touch in the age of Ebola. Nursing Outlook. 2015;63(1), 25-26. Doi: 10.1016/j.outlook.2014.11.016

[17] Downes, E: Nursing and complex humanitarian emergencies- Ebola is more than a disease. Nursing Outlook. 2015;63(1), 12-15. doi: 10.1016/j.outlook.2014.11.010

[18] World Health Organization factsheet. Avian Influenza. n.d. Available from: http://www.who.int/topics/avian_influenza/en/ [Accessed: 2018-04-11]

[19] World Health Organization factsheet. Cholera. n.d. Available from: http://www.who.int/mediacentre/factsheets/fs107/en/[Accessed: 2018-04-11]

[20] Centers for Disease Control and Prevention. Yellow fever. 2015. Available from: https://www.cdc.gov/yellowfever/index.html [Accessed: 2018-04-11]

[21] World Health Organization factsheet. Middle East Respiratory Syndrome Coronavirus. 2018. Available from: http://www.who.int/mediacentre/factsheets/mers-cov/en/ [Accessed: 2018-04-11]

[22] World Health Organization factsheet. Marburg disease. 2017. Available from: http://www.who.int/mediacentre/factsheets/fs_marburg/en/ [Accessed: 2018-04-11]

[23] World Health Organization factsheet. Zika virus infection. 2016. Available from: http://www.who.int/mediacentre/factsheets/zika/en/[Accessed: 2018-04-11]

[24] Centers for Disease Control and Prevention. Zika virus disease. 2016. Available from: https://www.cdc.gov/zika/about/index.html [Accessed: 2018-04-11]

[25] World Health Organization: Coronavirus, Available from: https://www.who.int/health-topics/coronavirus#tab=tab_1 [Accessed: 2020-12-02]

[26] Stratton, S.J: Ebola: Who is responsible for the political failure? Prehospital and Disaster Medicine. 2014;29(6), 553-554.

[27] Marshall, K. & Smith, S: Religion and Ebola: Learning from experience. Lancet. 2015; e25–e25. Doi:10.1016/s0140-6736(15)61082-0

Section 3

Midwives in Society

Chapter 8

The Impact of Antenatal Care in Maternal and Perinatal Health

Teketel Ermias Geltore and Dereje Laloto Anore

Abstract

Every moment, somewhere in our planet especially in low in come country, women of reproductive age group die from problems linked to gestations. The major reason for this enormous magnitude of complication is failure to use antenatal care services particularly in developing countries. The World Health Organization recommends a minimum of four ANC visits. However, global estimates indicate that only about half of all pregnant women receive this recommended amount of care. Antenatal care is one of the evidence-based interventions to decrease the probability of bad health outcomes for mothers and their newborns. Effectiveness of antenatal care, however, relies on the quality of care provided during each antenatal care visits. Antenatal care is an umbrella term used to describe the medical procedures and care that carried out starting from preconception. It is a care a woman receives throughout her pregnancy and is important in helping to ensure a healthy pregnancy state and safe childbirth. Therefore, antenatal care is to assure that every wanted pregnancy results in the delivery of a healthy baby without impairing the mother's health. The aim of this chapter is to examine the impact of antenatal care in decreasing maternal and newborn death from preconception through postnatal period.

Keywords: ANC Care, impact of ANC, preconception

1. Introduction

The World Health Organization launched a safe motherhood initiative in 1987, which aimed to reduce the number of complications and deaths related with pregnancy and childbirth [1]. In the provision of prenatal care, service care providers have often under emphasized women's health and health interventions aimed at improving reproductive care [2].

Healthy lifestyles during pregnancy are known to be associated with improved pregnancy outcomes for both mothers and offspring. As such, much attention has been placed on designing effective prenatal care guidance, and considerable research has been done to identify appropriate interventions to improve maternal and child health during the prenatal period [3, 4].

Among women who become pregnant, health risks experienced in the preconception period often continue during pregnancy, such as the use of alcohol, tobacco and other substances. Furthermore, the increasing prevalence of obesity and chronic conditions demand attention in the context of preconception care [5]. If these factors are not managed properly during this period, they may result in preterm delivery, low birth weight, stillbirth, birth defects, abortion and maternal complication [6–11].

IntechOpen

Antenatal care is a comprehensive health supervision of a pregnant woman before delivery or it is planned examination, observation and guidance given to the pregnant women from preconception until postnatal period. The antenatal period presents an important chance for detecting threats to the mother and unborn baby's health, as well as for counseling on nutrition, danger signs, and family planning options after the birth [12, 13].

To reduce maternal and neonatal morbidity and mortality, the World Health Organization recommended that pregnant women should receive ANC services at least 4 times starting from the first trimester of pregnancy [14–16].

Good ANC for pregnant women has become a vital component in the safe motherhood program whose aim is to improve the outcome of pregnancy for mother and newborn [17, 18].

According to the WHO report, 60 million deliveries take place globally each year in which the woman is cared for her by relatives only, or by no one at all. Being a long distance from health services, multiple demands for women's time, low coverage and poor quality of ANC have been identified as key factors [19, 20].

In addition to the risk of dying during pregnancy and childbirth, many more women suffer from short and long-term maternal disabilities and illness. According to WHO for every maternal death, an estimated 30 to 50 women suffer pregnancy related health problems such as vesico vaginal fistulae, infertility, and depression that can be permanently debilitating [21].

ANC provides possibility to provide pregnant women with information, treat existing social and medical conditions, as well as screen for risk factors. However, it is not enough to receive ANC, because majority of the fatal complications occur during or shortly after delivery. Therefore, availability of skilled obstetric attendance during delivery is mandatory. However, use of these services in most developing countries is inhibited due to various cultural and demographic factors. As the result, disproportions between high income and low-income countries regarding use ANC, labor and delivery as well as postpartum services showed many difference. In developed countries about 97% of the pregnant women receive ANC and 99% use trained personnel during delivery, whereas in developing countries, only 65% and 53% of women use ANC and skilled obstetric care services, respectively [22, 23]. The aim of this chapter is to provide information on the importance of antenatal care in decreasing maternal and newborn death from preconception through postnatal period. This chapter identified the risk factors are associated with negative health outcomes for the woman, her fetus.

2. The benefits of ANC in decreasing maternal and neonatal death

According to the studies conducted in different countries, the finding revealed that provision of 0.4 mg of folic acid three months prior to pregnancy, during pregnancy, and six weeks postpartum has been associated with more than 80% reduction in different types of specific congenital anomalies [24–31]. On the other hand, the finding of different studies showed that preconception folic acid administration is associated with increased fetal growth, and decreased risks of low birth weight [32–34]. Moreover, other study result depicted that the consumption of folic acid prior to conception can decrease the risk of developing anemia [35].

The provision of ANC services brings with it a positive impact and it can be achieved through screening for pregnancy problems, assessing risk factors, treating problems that may arise during the antenatal period, providing information to the pregnant woman, preparing physically and psychologically for parturition and parenthood [36–38].

Moreover, it also focuses on educating the pregnant woman on a range of topics, including well-being, birth preparedness, complication readiness, and breastfeeding [39, 40]. ANC also provides effective interventions for preventing and treating certain conditions, such as anemia, hypertensive disorders of pregnancy, sexually transmitted diseases including HIV/AIDS external cephalic version to detect a breeched position [39, 41, 42]. The overall aim of ANC is to produce a healthy mother and baby at the end of pregnancy by allocating necessary budgetary resource [43–45]. The recommended time for patients to receive ANCIS; first visit better before or at 16 weeks, with the next visit at 24 and 28 weeks, third visit at 30–32 weeks and fourth visit better from 36 to 40 weeks. During these visits, the healthcare professional measures uterine height, checks fetal heartbeat, tests urine, and measures the mother's blood pressure [40].

ANC indirectly saves the lives of mothers and babies by promoting and establishing good health before childbirth and the early postnatal period — the periods of highest risk. ANC often presents the first contact opportunity for a woman to connect with health services, thus offering an entry point for integrated care, promoting healthy home practices, influencing care seeking behaviors, and linking women with pregnancy complications to a referral system. Women are more likely to give with a skilled attendant if they have had at least one ANC visit [46].

ANC offers pregnant women chance to access protectiv'e care. In dev'eloping countries where access to emergency obstetric services is limited, ANC presents a viable option for pregnant women to be screened for potential risks during pregnancy or delivery. lt also provides an opportunity for treatment and health education including nutritional advice. On one hand practice of ANC, including the number of visits, to be associated with reduced risk of neonatal mortality, On the other hand, others study findings showed that found adverse or no relations between ANC utilization and birth outcomes and insufficient evidence that ANC interventions reduced neonatal or infant mortality in vulnerable populations [47–51].

ANC is very important in detection of high-risk pregnancies through the analysis of socioeconomic, medical and obstetrical factors. Beside to this, it is used as a platform for additional interventions that have been shown to positively influence the maternal and child health status, such as immunization, nutrition programs, breastfeeding and family planning and birth spacing counseling. Furthermore, ANC programs are used to provide care and information that is not directly related to pregnancy but can reduce the possible maternal risk factors, such as promoting healthy lifestyles, tackle malnutrition or inform about gender-based violence [52–70].

Some studies finding showed that ANC from a skilled provider was associated with decreased risk of neonatal mortality by the provision of the most effective ANC interventions included TT injection, and weight and blood pressure measurements [71].

TT vaccination that provide during ANC, protects the mother and the baby against tetanus, a deadly infection caused by Clostridium tetani bacteria, which enter the body through skin cuts and wounds such as those during delivery or cutting of the umbilical cord [72, 73].

In high-income settings, provision of ANC, skillful midwife-led has been associated with positive outcomes, including fewer preterm births, fewer fetal losses at any gestation, and high rates of positive experiences reported by women [74].

To improve maternal, newborn, and child health, the World Health Organization and other organizations, over the past years, have been encouraging for continuum of care. lt can provide as a key package of programs for MNCH, and can show a corridor to help reduce maternal and neonatal deaths [75–78].

Effective and timely maternal health care before conception, as well as during pregnancy and childbirth, could save nearly 3 million newborns in high burden countries. Most neonatal deaths could be prevented by direct interventions. Evidence suggests that two thirds of neonatal deaths could be prevented if all pregnant mothers and newborns had access to cost-effective and direct interventions as well as receiving care from skilled health care providers during pregnancy and childbirth [79–88].

High quality ANC can also influence women's health seeking behavior towards choosing skilled care at birth and helping them prepare to be able to access it. A positive experience during both pregnancy and childbirth are vital to person-centered care and the right of every childbearing woman, as highlighted in recent World Health Organization recommendations [89–94].

3. Risk factors are associated with negative health outcomes for the woman, her fetus

A literature review reported usage of ginger during pregnancy is not a safe. Higher doses of ginger can cause thinning of blood, stomach discomfort and heartburn [95–99].

In developing countries, child marriage is widespread, with almost one-third of girls being married before age 18. A practice that is driven by poverty, social norms, and discrimination against girls, child marriage has emerged as an important social issue in recent years, due in part to increased concerns among reproductive health advocates about the harmful consequences for young women marrying too early. As a result: dropping out of school; health risks that result from early sexual activity and pregnancy, including sexually transmitted diseases and maternal mortality; being prevented from taking advantage of economic opportunities; and if they have children, child malnutrition and mortality. Moreover, at child marriage deprives girls of their basic human rights and puts them at risk for harmful practices including exploitation, intimate partner violence, and abuse [100–103].

A study conducted in Italy, and the result exposures of women to chemical agents, pesticides, physical agents, ergonomic factors and stress, it appears that at present the evidence is sufficient to warrant the maximum protection of pregnant women to several well-documented occupational risk factors. These include exposures to anaesthetic gases, antineoplastic drugs, heavy metals, solvents, heavy physical work and irregular work schedules. For other work risks, such as exposure to nonionizing radiation and psychosocial work stress, the evidence is often suggestive but not conclusive [104].

Substance use during pregnancy can be risky to the woman's health and that of her children in both the short and long term. Most drugs, including opioids and stimulants, could potentially harm an unborn baby. Use of some substances can increase the risk of miscarriage and can cause migraines, seizures, or high blood pressure in the mother, which may affect her fetus. In addition, the risk of stillbirth is 2 to 3 times greater in women who smoke tobacco or marijuana, take prescription pain relievers, or use illegal drugs during pregnancy [105]. Smoking tobacco during pregnancy is estimated to have caused 1,015 infant deaths per year from 2005 through 2009 [106].

Anemia during pregnancy is an important factor for negative health outcome for mother and her new born. The causes of anemia during pregnancy in developing countries are multifactorial; these include micronutrient deficiencies of iron, folate, and vitamins A and B12 and anemia due to parasitic infections such as malaria and hookworm or chronic infections like TB and HIV [107–111].

4. Conclusion

Antenatal care is an important determinant of high maternal mortality rate and one of the basic components of maternal care on which the life of mothers and babies depend. Thus, Antenatal care is a key strategy to improve maternal and infant health.

Early initiation of antenatal care facilitates the timely management and treatment of pregnancy complications to reduce maternal and newborns deaths.

Studies examining the effectiveness of antenatal care on maternal and newborn health outcomes have provided conflicting results.

Good ANC links the woman and her family with the formal health system, increases the chance of using a skilled attendant at birth and contributes to good health through the life cycle. Inadequate care during this time breaks a critical link in the continuum of care, and affects both women and babies.

Indirect causes of maternal morbidity and mortality, such as HIV and malaria infections, contribute to approximately 25% of maternal deaths and near misses, so that by utilization of appropriate ANC services STIs and other diseases can be prevented and managed concurrently through integrated service delivery.

Author details

Teketel Ermias Geltore[1]* and Dereje Laloto Anore[2]

1 Midwifery Department, School of Nursing and Midwifery, College of Health Sciences and Medicine, Wachemo University–Durame Campus, Durame, Ethiopia

2 KembataTembaro Zone Health Department, Durame, Ethiopia

*Address all correspondence to: teketelermias@gmail.com

References

[1] Patel BB, Gurmeet P, Sinalkar DR, Pandya KH, Mahen A, Singh N. A study on knowledge and practices of antenatal care among pregnant women attending antenatal clinic at a Tertiary Care Hospital of Pune, Maharashtra. Med J DY PatilUniv 2016; 9:354-362.

[2] Atrash H, Jack BW, Johnson K, Coonrod DV, Moos M-K, Stubblefield PG, et al. Where is the "W"oman in MCH? Am J ObstetGynecol 2008; 199(6, Suppl. B): S259-65.

[3] Chapin RE, Robbins WA, Schieve LA, Sweeney AM, Tabacova SA, Tomashek KM: Off to a good start: the influence of pre- and periconceptional exposures, parental fertility, and nutrition on child's health. Environ Health Perspect 2004, 112:69-78.

[4] Association of state public health nutritionists; Preconception health: The role of nutrition. 2015

[5] Begum KS, Sachchithanantham K, De Somsubhra S. Maternal obesity and pregnancy outcome. Clin Exp ObstetGynecol 2010; 38(1):14-20.

[6] World Health Organization. Preconception health Regional expert group consultation on preconception care, in New Delhi, India. 2013

[7] Curtis M, Abelman S, Schulkin J, Williams JL, Fassett EM (2006) The History of preconception care: Evolving guidelines and standards. Maternal Child Health 10: 43-52.

[8] Hanson MA, Bardsley A, De-Regil LM, Moore SE, Oken E, et al. The International Federation of Gynecology and Obstetrics (FIGO) recommendations on adolescent, preconception, and maternal nutrition. Int J Gynecol Obstet. 2015 131: S213-S253.

[9] Centre for disease control. Control and prevention of rubella: evaluation and management of suspected outbreaks, rubella in pregnant women, and surveillance for congenital rubella syndrome. MMWR 50: 23.

[10] Hoyt MJ, Storm DS, Aaron E, Anderson J Preconception and contraceptive care for women living with HIV. Infectious Diseases in Obstetrics and Gynecology. 2012 P: 604183.

[11] Cruz J, Márquez A, Lang J, Valdés L Care to pregnancy diabetic achievement and challenge in Cuba. Sci FLO public health. 2013 15: 3.

[12] World Health Organization (WHO). What is the effectiveness of antenatal care? Copenhagen, WHO Regional Office for Europe, Health Evidence Network report; accessed. March 23, 2009. Website available at http://www.euro.who.int/Document/ E879 97.pdf,

[13] Carroli G, Rooney C, Villar J. How effective is antenatal care in preventing maternal mortality and serious morbidity? An overview of the evidence. Paediatr Perinat Epidemiol. 2001; 15(Supply 1):1-42.

[14] J. Villar and B. Bergsjo, UNDP/UNFPA/WHO/World Bank Special Program of Research, Development and Research Training in Human Reproduction. WHO Antenatal Care Randomized Trial: Manual for the Implementation of the New Model, World Health Organization-Department of Reproductive Health and Research, Geneva, Switzerland, 2002.

[15] World health organization Preconception care: Maximizing the gains for maternal and child health. Global consensus meeting. 2012

[16] World health organization Reduction of maternal and child

mortality and morbidity. What´s the role of Preconception care in the life course approach. Third congress on preconception health and care, Uppsala, Sweden. 2016

[17] Omigbodun AO. Preconception and antenatal care. In: Comprehensive Obstetrics in the Tropics. Ch 2. Kwawukume EY, Emuveyan EE, eds. Accra: Asante and Hittscher, 2002:7-14

[18] Yakoob MY, Menezes EV, Soomro T, Haws RA, Darmstadt GL, Bhutta ZA. Reducing stillbirths: behavioural and nutritional interventions before and during pregnancy. BMC Pregnancy Childbirth 2009;9:10

[19] Darmstadt GL, Lee AC, Cousens S, Sibley L, Bhutta ZA, Donnay F, Osrin D, Bang A, Kumar V, Wall SN, Baqui A, Lawn JE: 60 million non-facility births: who can deliver in community settings to reduce intra-partum related deaths? Int J Gynaecol Obstet 2009, 107: S89–S112.

[20] Mrisho M, Schellenberg JA, Mushi AK, Obrist B, Mshinda H, Tanner M, Schellenberg D: Factors affecting home delivery in rural Tanzania. Trop Med Int Health 2007, 12:862-872.

[21] WHO, Maternal Mortality in 1995: Estimates Developed by WHO, UNICEF, UNFPA and the World Bank, WHO, Geneva, Switzerland, 2001.

[22] I. Addai, "Determinants of use ofmaternal-child health services in rural Ghana," Journal of Biosocial Science, vol. 32, no. 1, pp. 1– 15, 2000.

[23] Family Care International and the Safe Motherhood Inter Agency Group, 2002, http://www.safemotherhood.org/.

[24] T. Marchant, J.A. Schellenberg, R. Nathanetal. "Anemia in pregnancy and infant mortality in Tanzania," Tropical Medicine and International Health, vol. 9, no. 2, pp.262-266, 2004.

[25] F. Habib, E. H. Alabdin, M. Alenazy, and R. Nooh, "Compliance to iron supplementation during pregnancy," Journal of Obstetrics and Gynecology, vol. 29, no. 6, pp. 487-492, 2009.

[26] E. Ekweagwu, A. E. Agwu, and E. Madukwe, "The role of micronutrients in child health: are views of literature, "African Journal of Biotechnology, vol. 7, no. 11, pp.1604-1611, 2008.

[27] D. K. Tobias, C. Z. hang, J. Chavarro et al., "Pre pregnancy adherence to dietary patterns and lower risk of gestational diabetes mellitus," American Journal of Clinical Nutrition, vol. 96, no. 2, pp. 289-295, 2012.

[28] A. Czeizel, M. Dob´ o, and P. Vargha, "Hungarian cohort controlled trial of pre conception multivitamin supplementation shows a reduction in certain congenital abnormalities," Birth Defects Research Part A: Clinical and Molecular Teratology, vol. 70, no. 11, pp. 853-861, 2004

[29] M. K. Moos, "Pre conception health promotion: progress in changing a prevention paradigm," Journal of Perinatal & Neonatal Nursing, vol. 12, no. 78, pp. 2-13, 2004.

[30] G. Teckie, A. Kromberg, and J. G. R Kromberg, "Neural tube defects in Gauteng, South Africa: recurrence risks and associated factors," South African Medical Journal, vol. 103, no. 12, pp. 973-977, 2013.

[31] M. Viswanathan, K. A. Treiman, J. Doto, J. C. Middleton, E. J. L. Coker-Schwimmer, and W. K. Nicholson, "Folic acid supplementation for the prevention of neural tube defects," JAMA, vol. 2017, no. 317, p. 2, 2015.

[32] V. A. Hodgetts, R. K. Morris, A. Francis, J. Gardosi, and K. M. Ismail,

"Effectiveness of folic acid supplementation in pregnancy on reducing the risk of small-for-gestational age neonates: a population study, systematic review and met analysis," BJOG: An International Journal of Obstetrics & Gynecology, vol. 122, no. 4, pp. 478-490, 2014.

[33] S. Timmermans, V. Jaddoe, A. Hofmannsthal., "Preconception folic acid supplementation, fetal growth and the risks of low birth weight and preterm birth: the Generation R Study," British Journalof Nutrition, vol. 102,no.5,pp. 777-785, 200

[34] B.O. Verburg, E.A. Steegers, M.DeRidderetal. "New charts for ultrasound dating of pregnancy and assessment of fetal growth: longitudinal data from a population-based cohort study, "Ultrasound in Obstetrics and Gynecology, vol. 31, no. 4, pp. 388-396, 2008.

[35] J. A. Greenberg, S. J. Bell, Y. Guan, and Y. H. Yu, "Folic acid supplementation and pregnancy: more than just neural tube defect prevention," Reviews in Obstetrics & Gynecology, vol. 4, no. 5, pp. 2-9, 2011.

[36] Kisuule I, Kaye DK, Najjuka F, et al. Timing and reasons for coming late for the first antenatal care visit by pregnant women at Mulago hospital, Kampala Uganda. BMC Preg Childbirth. 2013; 13:1.

[37] Perumal N, Cole DC, Ouédraogo HZ, et al. Health andnutrition knowledge, attitudes and practices of pregnantwomen attending and not-attending ANC clinics in Western Kenya: a cross-sectional analysis. BMC Preg Childbirth. 2013; 13:1.

[38] WHO Global Health Observatory (GHO): Antenatal caresituationsand trends. 2011.

[39] Das AC. A comprehensive study on the effectiveness of voucher scheme on antenatal, delivery and postnatal care among poor women in Bhola District, Bangladesh. Int J Higher Edu Res 2015; 5(2):1-11.

[40] Ministry of Health Report. Memorandum on antenatal clinics: their conduct and scope. Ministry of Health, London, 1929.

[41] Maine D. Safe motherhood programs: options and issues. Prevention of maternal mortality. Center for Population and Family Health. United States of America, 1991.

[42] Das AC. exploring the constraints regarding maternal health in reproductive age among the rural women in Bangladesh. Mediscope 2016; 3(2):1-10.

[43] Lucas AO, Stoll BJ, Bale JR. Improving birth outcomes: meeting the challenge in the developing world. National Academies Press; 2003.

[44] Lindmark G, Cnattingius S. The scientific basis of antenatal care: report from a state-of-the-art conference. Acta ObstetGynecolScand 1991; 70(2):105-109.

[45] Gay J, Hardee K, Judice N, et al. What works: a policy and program guide to the evidence on family planning, safe motherhood and STI/HIV/AIDS Interventions: Module 1: Safe Motherhood. POLICY Project, 2003

[46] Ornella Lincetto, Seipati Mothebesoane-Anoh, Patricia Gomez, Stephen Munjanja. Opportunities for Africa's Newborns

[47] Ibrahim J, Yorifuji T, Tsuda T, Kashima S, Doi H. Frequency of antenatal care visits and neonatal mortality in Indonesia. J Trop Pediatr 2012; 58:184-188.

[48] Raatikainen K, Heiskanen N, Heinonen S. Under-attending free antenatal care is associated with adverse pregnancy outcomes. BMC Public Health 2007;7:1.

[49] . Hollowell J, Oakley L, Kurinczuk JJ, Brocklehurst P, Gray R. The effectiveness of antenatal care programs to reduce infant mortality and preterm birth in socially disadvantaged and vulnerable women in high-income countries: a systematic review. BMC Pregnancy Childbirth 2011; 11:13.

[50] Singh A, Pallikadavath S, Ram F, Alagarajan M. Do antenatal care interventions improve neonatal survival in India? Health Policy Plan 2014; 29:842-848.

[51] Dowswell T, Carroli G, Duley L et al. Alternative versus standard packages of antenatal care for low-risk pregnancy. Cochrane Database Syst Rev. 2010; 10:CD000934.

[52] Imdad A, Bhutta ZA. Effects of calcium supplementation during pregnancy on maternal, fetal and birth outcomes. Paediatr Perinat Epidemiol2012; 26Suppl 1:138-52.

[53] Oddy WH, Kendall GE, Li J, et al. The long-term effects of breastfeeding on child and adolescent mental health: a pregnancy cohort study followed for 14 years. J Pediatr 2010; 156:568-574.

[54] Black RE, Victora CG, Walker SP, et al. Maternal and child under nutrition and overweight in low-income and middle-income countries. Lancet 2013; 382:427-451.

[55] Gupta A. Breastfeeding and child health. Economic and Political Weekly 2006.

[56] Ota E, Hori H, Mori R, et al. Antenatal dietary education and supplementation to increase energy and protein intake. Cochrane Database Systematic Review. 2015.

[57] . Pena-Rosas JP, De-Regil LM, Garcia-Casal MN, et al. Daily oral iron supplementation during pregnancy. Cochrane Database Systematic Review. 2015.

[58] Haider BA, Bhutta ZA. Multiple-micronutrient supplementation for women during pregnancy. Cochrane Database Systematic Review 2015.

[59] . World Health Organization. WHO statement on antenatal care. Geneva, Switzerland: World Health Organization, 2011

[60] McNellan CR, Dansereau E, Colombara D, et al. Uptake of antenatal care, and its relationship with participation in health services and behaviors: an analysis of the poorest regions of four Mesoamerican countries. Ann Glob Health 2017; 83:193-194.

[61] Chen XK, Wen SW, Yang Q, et al. Adequacy of prenatal care and neonatal mortality in infants born to mothers with and without antenatal high-risk conditions. Aust N Z J Obstet Gynaecol2007; 47:122-7.

[62] Zanconato G, Msolomba R, Guarenti L, et al. Antenatal care in developing countries: the need for a tailored model. Semin Fetal Neonatal Med 2006; 11:15-20.

[63] PMNCH. The PMNCH Report 2012. Analysing Progress on Commitments to the Global Strategy for Women's and Children's Health. Geneva, Switzerland: World Health Organization, 2012.

[64] Titaley CR, Dibley MJ. Antenatal iron/folic acid supplements, but not postnatal care, prevents neonatal deaths in Indonesia: analysis of Indonesia demographic and health surveys 2002/2003-2007 (a retrospective cohort study). BMJ Open 2012;2:e001399

[65] deJongh TE, Gurol-Urganci I, Allen E, et al. Integration of antenatal care services with health programmes in low- and middle-income countries: systematic review. J Glob Health 2016; 6:010403.

[66] Abou-Zahr C, Wardlaw T. Antenatal care in developing countries: promises, achievements and missed opportunities. Geneva: World Health Organization, 2003.

[67] Khan KS, Wojdyla D, Say L, et al. WHO analysis of causes of maternal death: a systematic review. Lancet 2006; 367:1066-1074.

[68] Lincetto O, Mothebesoane-Anoh S, Gomez P, et al. In opportunities for Africa's newborns. PMNCH 2006.

[69] Carroli G, Rooney C, Villar J. How effective is antenatal care in preventing maternal mortality and serious morbidity? An overview of the evidence. Paediatr Perinat Epidemiol2001;15Suppl 1:1-42.

[70] Moss W, Darmstadt GL, Marsh DR, et al. Research priorities for the reduction of perinatal and neonatal morbidity and mortality in

[71] McCurdy RJ, Kjerulff KH, Zhu J. Prenatal care associated with reduction of neonatal mortality in Sub-Saharan Africa: evidence from Demographic and Health Surveys. Acta ObstetGynecol Scand. 2011; 90:779-790.

[72] World Health Organization. Maternal immunization against tetanus: integrated management of pregnancy and childbirth. Geneva: World Health Organization; 2006.

[73] Demicheli V, Barale A, Rivetti A. Vaccines for women for preventing neonatal tetanus. Cochrane Database Syst Rev. 2015; 7:Cd002959.

[74] Sandall J, Soltani H, Gates S, Shennan A, Devane D. Midwifery-led continuity models versus other models of care for childbearing women. Cochrane Database Syst Rev 2016;4: CD004667.

[75] Tinker A, ten Hoope-Bender P, Azfar S, Bustreo F, Bell R. A continuum of care to save newborn lives. The Lancet. 2005; 365: 822-825.

[76] Kerber KJ, de Graft-Johnson JE, Bhutta ZA, Okong P, Starrs A, Lawn JE. Continuum of care for maternal, newborn, and child health: from slogan to service delivery. The Lancet. 2007; 370: 1358-1369.

[77] Martines J, Paul VK, Bhutta ZA, Koblinsky M, Soucat A, Walker N, et al. Neonatal survival: a call for action. Lancet. 2005; 365: 1189-1197.doi: 10.1016/S0140-6736(05)71882-1 PMID: 15794974

[78] UNICEF, UNICEF. Committing to Child Survival Progress Report 2012: a Promise Renewed.[Internet]. New York: United Nations Children's Fund, The (UNICEF); 2012. Available: http://www.unicef.org/ publications/files/APR_Progress_Report_2012_11Sept2012.pdf

[79] Black RE, Cousens S, Johnson HL, Lawn JE, Rudan I, Bassani DG, et al. Global, regional, and national causes of child mortality in 2008: a systematic analysis. Lancet. 2010; 375(9730):1969-87. https://doi.org/10.1016/S0140-6736(10)60549-1 PMID: 20466419

[80] Liu L, Johnson HL, Cousens S, Perin J, Scott S, Lawn JE, et al. Global, regional, and national causes of child mortality: an updated systematic analysis for 2010 with time trends since 2000. Lancet. 2012; 379 (9832):2151-61. https://doi.org/10.1016/S0140-6736(12)60560-1 PMID: 22579125

[81] Lawn J, Kerber K. Opportunities for Africas newborns: practical data policy and programmatic support for newborn care in Africa. 2006.

[82] Darmstadt GL, Walker N, Lawn JE, Bhutta ZA, Haws RA, Cousens S. Saving newborn lives in Asia and Africa: cost and impact of phased scale-up of interventions within the continuum of care. Health policy and planning. 2008; 23(2):101-17. https://doi.org/10.1093/heapol/czn001PMID: 18267961

[83] Unicef. Committing to child survival: a promise renewed. Progress report 2015.New York: UNICEF. 2015.

[84] Bhutta ZA, Das JK, Bahl R, Lawn JE, Salam RA, Paul VK, et al. Can available interventions end preventable deaths in mothers, newborn babies, and stillbirths, and at what cost? The Lancet. 2014; 384 (9940):347-370.

[85] UNICEF. Levels & trends in child mortality. Estimates developed by the UN inter-agency group for child mortality estimation. New York: UNICEF. 2017.

[86] WHO. Every Newborn: An action plan to end preventable deaths. 2014.

[87] UN DoEaSA, Population Division, Population Division. World population prospects: The 2015 Revision, Key Findings and Advance Tables. Working Paper No. ESA/P/WP. 241; 2015

[88] Raven JH, Tolhurst RJ, Tang S, Van Den Broek N. What is quality in maternal and neonatal health care? Midwifery. 2012; 28(5):e676–e83. https://doi.org/10.1016/j.midw.2011.09.003 PMID: 22018395

[89] WHO | WHO statement on antenatal care. WHO.http://www.who.int/maternal_child_adolescent/documents/rhr_11_12/en/. Accessed 9 Sep 2013.

[90] Chukwuma A, Wosu AC, Mbachu C, Weze K. Quality of antenatal care predicts retention in skilled birth attendance: a multilevel analysis of 28 African countries. BMC Pregnancy Childbirth. 2017;17:152.

[91] Adjiwanou V, LeGrand T. Does antenatal care matter in the use of skilled birth attendance in rural Africa: a multi-country analysis? SocSci Med. 2013; 86:26-34.

[92] Afulani PA, Moyer C. Explaining disparities in use of skilled birth attendants in developing countries: a conceptual framework. PLoS One. 2016; 11:0154110.

[93] World Health Organisation. WHO recommendations on antenatal care for a positive pregnancy experience. 2016. http://www.who.int/reproductivehealth/publications/maternal_perinatal_health/anc-positivepregnancy- experience/en/. Accessed 18 Sep 2018.

[94] World Health Organization. WHO recommendations: intrapartum care for a positive childbirth experience. WHO. 2018. http://www.who.int/reproductivehealth/ publications/intrapartum-care-guidelines/en/. Accessed 28 Feb 2018.

[95] Tunçalp Ö, Were W, MacLennan C, Oladapo O, Gülmezoglu A, Bahl R, et al. Quality of care for pregnant women and newborns—the WHO vision. BJOGInt J ObstetGynaecol. 2015; 122:1045-1049.

[96] Loke Y, editor. Pregnancy and Breastfeeding Medicines Guide. 1st ed. Melbourne: The Royal Women's Hospital, Pharmacy Department; 2010

[97] Braun L, Cohen M. Herbsand Natural Supplements. Third ed. Churchill Livingstone, Australia: Elsevier; 2010

[98] Australian Pharmaceutical Formulary and Handbook. 22nd ed. Canberra: Pharmaceutical Society of Australia; 2012

[99] Wilkinson JM. What do we know about herbal morning sickness treatments? A literature survey. Midwifery. 2000; 16:224-228

[100] UNICEF. State of the World's Children 2013: Children with Disabilities. New York: United Nations Children's Fund; 2013.

[101] Mensch BS, Singh S, Casterline JB. Trends in the timing of first marriage among men and women in the developing world.In: Lloyd CB, Behrman JR, Stromquist NP, Cohen B, editors. The changing transitions to adulthood in developing countries: Selected studies. Washington, D.C.: The National Academies Press; 2006. p. 118-71.

[102] . Klugman J, Hanmer L, Twigg S, Hasan T, McCleary-Sills J, Santamaria J. Voice and Agency: Empowering Woman and Girls for Shared Prosperity. Washington DC: The World Bank Group; 2014.

[103] Jain S, Kurz K. New insights on preventing child marriage: A global analysis of factors and programs. New Delhi: International Center for Research on Women; 2007.

[104] Irene Figa`-Talamanca, Occupational risk factors and reproductive health of women Occupational Medicine 2006;56:521-531 doi:10.1093/occmed/kql114

[105] Tobacco, drug use in pregnancy can double risk of stillbirth. Eunice Kennedy Shriver National Institute of Child Health and Human Development. https://www.nichd.nih.gov/news/releases/Pages/121113-stillbirth-drug-use.aspx. Published December 11, 2013. Accessed January 31, 2018.

[106] National Center for Chronic Disease Prevention and Health Promotion (US) Office on Smoking and Health. The Health Consequences of Smoking—50 Years of Progress: A Report of the Surgeon General. Atlanta (GA): Centers for Disease Control and Prevention (US); 2014. http://www.ncbi.nlm.nih.gov/books/NBK179276/.

[107] S. E. Msuya, T. H. Hussein, J. Uriyo, N. E. Sam, and B. Stray-Pedersen, "Anaemia among pregnant women in northern Tanzania: prevalence, risk factors and effect on perinatal outcomes.," Tanzania Journal of Health Research, vol. 13, no. 1, pp. 33-39, 2011.

[108] E. M.McClure, S.R. Meshnick, P. Mungai et al., "The association of parasitic infections in pregnancy and maternal and fetal anemia: a cohort study in coastal Kenya," PLOS Neglected Tropical Diseases, vol. 8, no. 2, Article ID e2724, 2014.

[109] O. T. Okube, W. Mirie, E. Odhiambo, W. Sabina, and M. Habtu, "Prevalence and Factors Associated with Anaemia among Pregnant Women AttendingAntenatal Clinic in the Second and Third Trimesters at Pumwani Maternity Hospital, Kenya," Open Journal of Obstetrics and Gynecology, vol. 06, no. 01, pp. 16-27, 2016.

[110] S. Brooker, P. J. Hotez, and D. A. P. Bundy, "Hookworm-related anaemia among pregnant women: a systematic review," PLOS Neglected Tropical Diseases, vol. 2, no. 9, article e291, 2008.

[111] S. Ononge, O. Campbell, and F. Mirembe, "Haemoglobin status and predictors of anaemia among pregnant women in Mpigi, Uganda," BMC Research Notes, vol. 7, no. 1, article no. 712, 2014.

Chapter 9

Antenatal Diagnosis of Congenital Anomalies on Ultrasound Screening

Callen Kwamboka Onyambu and Norah Mukiri Tharamba

Abstract

Congenital fetal anomalies contribute to the global burden of disease in children. Various screening programs have been used for antenatal screening of these anomalies. Screening targets low risk population and is usually done in the second trimester though some are done at the mother's first antenatal visit especially in resource constrained setting. Mother's who have had a previous pregnancy with congenital anomaly are given targeted elaborate screening. Early diagnosis of this anomalies can lead to early intervention and better outcomes. Diagnosis of the malformations also leads to clinical decision making on mode of delivery thereby avoiding birth related trauma to the mother and the baby. In case of lethal congenital anomalies early diagnosis aids in clinical decision making on the management of the pregnancy.

Keywords: Ultrasound screening, pregnancy, fetal anomalies, fetal well being

1. Introduction

According to the World Health Organization (WHO), the term congenital anomaly includes any morphological, functional, biochemical or molecular defects that may develop in the embryo and fetus that is present at birth, whether detected at that time or not [1].

Major congenital anomalies impair function or greatly interfere with cosmetic value.

They may be life threatening and therefore need immediate management. Major anomalies could have a negative impact on a child's well-being and development, if early corrective surgery is not done. Minor anomalies, on the other hand, may cause little or no functional effects. They do not cause distress in the newborn and hence there is no urgency for their correction in the neonatal period [2].

Congenital anomalies occur in 2–3% of all births and are an important cause of perinatal morbidity and mortality accounting for 20–30% of perinatal deaths.

In a study conducted by Nayab Alia in Madina Teaching Hospital, Faisalabad on gray scale ultrasound, antenatal prevalence of congenital anomalies was 29.75 per 1000 and 2.97% [3]. A similar study in Saudi Arabia showed the antenatal prevalence of congenital anomalies to be 27.96 per 1000. The median maternal age at diagnosis was 27.5 years and the median gestational age at diagnosis was 31 weeks [4].

IntechOpen

However, the actual numbers of these anomalies vary among different countries with prevalence of anomalies reported to be 2% in England and 1.49% in South Africa [5]. The reason for the regional difference of congenital anomalies might be attributed to variable factors, such as: maternal risk factors, environmental exposures, ecological, economical and ethnic factors [6, 7].

1.1 Pattern of congenital anomalies

The patterns of congenital anomalies may be different between regions and the actual numbers may vary significantly between countries [8]. In different countries, people have varied cultural and religious practices including exposure during antenatal period to various environmental factors. This may contribute to varied patterns of congenital anomalies. In some instances a common exposure to teratogenic factors or a hereditary condition with variable penetrance, may lead to high numbers of some anomalies, where severely affected individuals were not observed because of fetal/infant mortality [9]. Certain population groups are also regarded as "high risk groups" for congenital anomalies such as those living in heavily polluted industrial zones [10].

According to one study, frequency of congenital anomalies was more in males than females, with CNS anomalies being the most common. The anomalies were more common in gestation age of 29–32 weeks [11]. In a retrospective study of 200 cases of congenital anomalies carried out in Jos, Nigeria, the highest incidence was reported in the gastrointestinal system 61 cases. No association was found between the occurrences of the various congenital anomalies [12].

In yet another study conducted among South African live born neonates at Kalafong Hospital, Pretoria, in which the incidence of congenital anomalies was 11.87 per 1,000 live births, the most commonly affected system was the central nervous system (2.30 per 1,000 live births) [13].

1.2 Risk factors for congenital anomalies

According to WHO, approximately 50% of all congenital anomalies cannot be associated with a specific cause. However, there are some known risk factors which include socioeconomic factors with an estimated 94% of severe birth defects occurring in middle and low income countries. This is because mothers are more susceptible to macronutrient and micronutrient malnutrition and may also have increased exposure to agents that cause or increase the incidence of abnormal prenatal development, especially infection and alcohol. Other known factors are genetic and environmental factors [14, 15]. This is reaffirmed by a study that was conducted in Tanzania, that showed significant association between congenital anomalies and lack of periconceptional use of folic acid, maternal age above 35 years, exposure to pollutants and high birth order above [16].

Women with uterine anomalies have also been found to be at risk for particular CAs. In one study, the risk for some specific defects such as nasal hypoplasia, omphalocele, limb deficiencies, teratomas, and anencephaly was four times higher among offspring of mothers with a bicornuate uterus [17].

1.3 Ultrasound imaging IN congenital anomalies

Many congenital anomalies are identified prenatally on usual work up which includes detailed ultrasound and amniocentesis.

The diagnostic ability of ultrasound is well established by several studies with detection rate dependent on a number of factors which include the type of abnormality, sophistication of equipment and experience of operator [18]. In a study conducted by Shama Munim at Aga Khan University Hospital (AKUH), Karachi on the accuracy of ultrasound in the diagnosis of congenital abnormalities, antenatal ultrasound successfully diagnosed fetal abnormalities in 48.8% of cases and more than 90% Central Nervous system defects and renal abnormalities [18].

However, a 1997 Report of the Royal College of Obstetricians and Gynecologists Working Party on Ultrasound Screening for Fetal Abnormalities identified that one of the problems with screening scans was the variable way in which they were conducted because there are no clear guidelines about what should, or should not, be examined. In a multicenter study, comparison was made of the precision of sonographic examinations done before 24 weeks gestational age at tertiary ultrasound laboratories contrasted with nontertiary ones. All the institutions were amply furnished with up-to-date equipment and supported with didactic and practical in-service training as required. The study found global sensitivity for sonographically demonstrable fetal abnormalities was 35% in tertiary centers, significantly higher compared to 13% in community hospitals. This further emphasizes that operator experience, competence, and training are vital determinants [19].

Ultrasound imaging is now routinely used in most countries for the purpose of screening pregnancies for fetal malformations but modalities, reliability and value of such screening is controversial [14, 19].

Regarding the time in gestation at which sonographic screening should be done, it is worthy noting that majority of the structural abnormalities are increasingly detected with advancing gestation. In early pregnancy, it is possible to diagnose with confidence certain categories of fetal anomalies, such as anencephaly, which can be reliably demonstrated at 10–14 weeks gestational age [20]. In certain instances, omphalocele and extremity malformations are also detectable using sonography in the first trimester, whereas other structural defects, like urinary system anomalies, are demonstrable later in pregnancy. However, a routine anomaly scan should be performed between 18 and 22 weeks of gestation. This period compromises between dating the pregnancy and the timely detection of major congenital anomalies [21].

Ultrasound examination at 10–14 weeks includes measurement of nuchal translucency, which is the maximum thickness of the subcutaneous translucency between the skin and the soft tissue overlying the cervical spine of the fetus. An increased nuchal translucency is associated with aneuploidy and cardiac malformations [22].

Ultrasound at around 20–21 weeks is done to screen fetuses for morphological anomalies. The utility of second trimester sonographic scan for detection of chromosomal anomalies was first recommended in 1985 [23]. Chromosomal aberrations were increasingly found to be associated with certain ultrasound findings, including biometric parameters (e.g., shortened femur and humerus, pyelectasis, thickened nuchal fold, dilated ventricles, fetal growth retardation) and morphologic features.

Ultrasound is the main diagnostic tool in the prenatal detection of congenital anomalies. It allows examination of the external and internal anatomy of the fetus. Even though a number of women are at increased risk of fetal malformations, either as a result of family history or owing to exposure to teratogens like infection and some drugs, the great majority of fetal abnormaitlies arise in the low risk category. As a result, sonographic evaluation ought to be offered routinely to all pregnant mothers. This is typically performed at 18–23 weeks of gestation, and should be done to a high level of precision. The scan should comprise systematic evaluation of the fetus for the detection of any defects.

2. Systemic review of congenital anomalies on ultrasound

2.1 Central nervous system (CNS)

The frequency of central nervous system anomalies varies according to geographic area and race. It is approximately 1–2:1000 newborns. Survivors are often severely disabled, necessitating long-term care.

The fetal brain undergoes major developmental changes during pregnancy. At 7 weeks of gestation, a sonolucent region is demonstrable in the cranial pole representing the fluid-filled rhombencephalic vesicle. At 9 weeks, demonstration of the convoluted pattern of the three primary cerebral vesicles is possible. The most prominent structures from 11 weeks are the echogenic choroid plexuses which fill the lateral ventricles. In the early second trimester, the lateral ventricles and choroid plexuses decrease in size relative to the brain mass.

Effective ultrasound screening for CNS anomalies can be carried out by examination of two important axial planes through the fetal brain; the transventricular and transcerebellar planes. Therefore, familiarity with the normal appearance of the fetal brain in these planes and at different gestational ages is vital for prompt identification of congenital anomalies.

The transventricular plane is at the level of the ventricular atria, with the echogenic choroid plexus being the dominant landmark. Measurements of atrial diameter made perpendicular to the walls should not normally exceed 10 mm.

This plane is obtained by axial sonogram at the level of the cavum septum pellucidum and shows the lateral margins of the frontal horns, the medial and lateral limits of the posterior horns of the lateral ventricles, and the choroid plexuses. It is used for fetal biometrics and quantification of the ventricular width (**Figure 1**).

The second crucial axial plane is the transcerebellar plane, which allows the examination of the midbrain and posterior fossa. The anatomic landmarks are the inferior portion of the third ventricle and the cerebellar hemispheres, which are outlined by fluid in the cisterna magna. The normal cisterna magna measures 2 to 11 mm in width (**Figure 2**).

A small cisterna magna (<2 mm) suggests a Chiari II malformation. However, it may also occur in massive ventriculomegaly. A large cisterna magna (>11 mm) may be a normal variant (megacisterna magna) or indicate a variety of anomalies. These

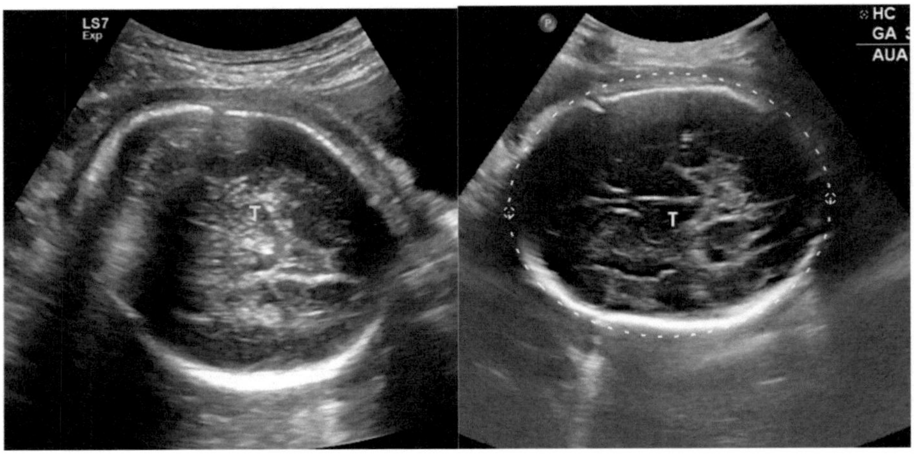

Figure 1.
Obstetric ultrasound showing biometric measurements. Fetal head: *Sonograms of the fetal head at the level of the thalami (T) showing measurement of the head circumference.*

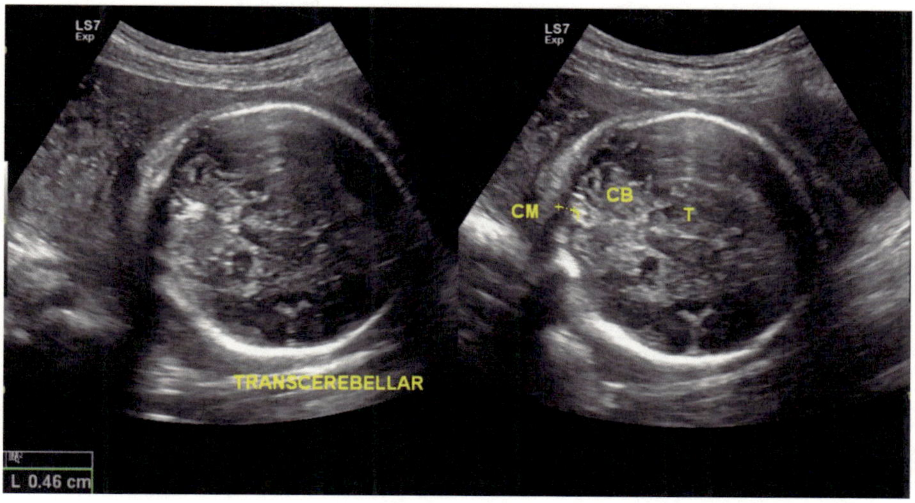

Figure 2.
Obstetric ultrasound; trans-cerebellar plane: This shows the cerebellar hemispheres (CB), cisterna magna (CM, between the two calibers) and thalami (T).

include Dandy-Walker malformation, arachnoid cyst, and cerebellar hypoplasia. When these two planes are anatomically normal, the risk of CNS anomaly is minute (0.005%).

Additional scanning planes along different orientations may be required occasionally, when one needs better definition of intracranial anatomy detail.

A sagittal and/or coronal view of the entire fetal spine should be obtained. In the sagittal plane, the normal spine has a 'double railway' appearance and one can appreciate intact soft tissue above it. In the coronal plane, the three ossification centers of the vertebra are visualized and should tether down into the sacrum. These views are used for assessment of vertebral integrity which rules out spina bifida. The presence and regularity of the whole spine from these views rules out sacral agenesis and scoliosis.

2.2 Cardiovascular system

The heart is the first functional organ in the embryo. It is prominently located and has visible contractions, which has made it the object of study for centuries. However, as recently as the late 1970s and early 1980s, the field of heart development was still in its infancy. In 1984, Dr. Constance Weinstein and colleagues at the National Institutes of Health (NIH) organized a meeting to bring together both cardiologists and basic scientists to summarize what was known about the development of the heart.

Congenital Heart Disease (CHD) is the most common birth defect comprising over 30 types of defects, ranging from mild to severe. It is found in 5–10 per 1,000 live births and in about 30 per 1,000 still births. Some forms of CHD resolve spontaneously, others are fully correctible, while others are life-threatening. Nearly 3 children out of every thousand live births have severe CHD requiring early surgery, while another 13/1000 requires surgery or catheter-based intervention later in childhood.

Precise US diagnosis of fetal heart abnormalities often requires specialized equipment and a high level of expertise.

The examination of the fetal heart begins with the assessment of the disposition of abdominal and thoracic organs. Abnormal disposition is associated with complex

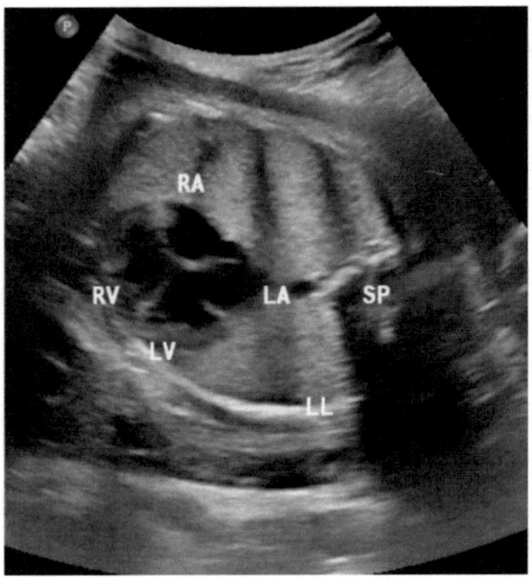

Figure 3.
Obstetric ultrasound; 4-chamber heart. Normal four-chamber view of the heart. Transverse scan through the fetal heart showing right ventricle (RV) anteriorly, left ventricle (LV) on the left, right atrium (RA) on the right and the left atrium (LA) as the most posterior. The spine (SP) and left lung (LL) are demonstrated.

cardiac anomalies. A transverse scan of the upper abdomen allows demonstration of the situation of the liver, stomach and great abdominal vessels. An axial section of the chest demonstration of a four-chamber view of the fetal heart. The heart covers about one third of the thorax. It is shifted to the left part of the thorax with the apex directed to the left.

About 90% of ultrasonographically detectable fetal cardiac defects demonstrate some abnormalities in the four-chamber view. Heart rate and rhythm are assessed subjectively. M-mode is useful for the evaluation of abnormal cases though is of little help in assessing morphology of the heart (**Figure 3**).

2.3 Pulmonary abnormalities

The lungs are interrogated in the same section used for the four-chamber view of the heart. The fetal lungs are uniformly echogenic. At 18–23 weeks, the middle third of the thoracic area at the level of the four-chamber view is occupied by the heart and the remaining two thirds by the lungs.

2.4 Anterior abdominal wall

The prevalence of anterior abdominal wall defects in sub Saharan Africa is not known as there are no population based studies. This could be due to non-availability of prenatal diagnosis and poor outcome of care post-delivery [24]. In a study carried out in a Nigerian tertiary hospital, omphalocele was the most common anterior abdominal wall defect seen [25].

Normal development of the anterior abdominal wall depends on the fusion of four folds (cephalic, caudal and two lateral). Developmental midgut herniation occurs at 8–10 weeks with subsequent retraction into the abdominal cavity at 10–12 weeks.

The integrity of the abdominal wall should always be adequately demonstrated. This is achieved via transverse scans which demonstrate the insertion of the umbilical cord. The urinary bladder should be visualized within the pelvis which rules out bladder exstrophy.

A study conducted to determine the ability of routine obstetric ultrasound to detect and accurately describe fetuses with anterior abdominal wall defects demonstrated examination between 16 and 22 weeks gestation detected 60% of defects with a false positive rate of 5.3%. Fetuses with gastroschisis were incorrectly assigned as exomphalos in 14.7% of cases recognized before 22 weeks gestation. The diagnosis was completely accurate in 71.6% of cases. Therefore, problems of diagnostic accuracy should be put into consideration when counseling couples with a fetal anomaly.

2.5 Gastrointestinal tract

The fetal abdomen differs from the abdomen of the older child or adult. The fetal abdomen is large in relation to its body dimension compared with the adult. The liver is larger with the left lobe is bigger than the right owing to its greater supply of oxygenated blood. The umbilical vein is an important US landmark. Half the blood it carries goes directly to the inferior vena cava via the ductus venosus. The remainder perfuses the liver via the left portal vein. The gall bladder is visualized as an ovoid cystic structure below the intrahepatic portion of the umbilical vein. The spleen may be demonstrated in a transverse plane posterior and to the left of the stomach. The adrenal glands are up to 20 times larger in relative size because of the presence of a fetal zone. The pelvis is small with the pelvic organs extending into the lower abdomen. Swallowing commences at 11 to 12 weeks gestational age (GA). The fetal stomach is visible from 9 weeks of gestation as a sonolucent cystic structure in the upper left quadrant of the abdomen. It should be filled with swallowed fluid by 18 weeks GA. The small bowel is moderately echogenic and centrally located. Peristalsis in small intestine loops is usually demonstrable by the third trimester. The visualized small gut usually measures just below 6 mm in width and below 15 mm in length. The large bowel is seen after 20 weeks of intrauterine life as a tubular organ in the periphery of the abdominal cavity. It gradually fills up with meconium but does not usually surpass 23 mm in caliber.

The abdominal circumference should be measured in a scan of the abdomen demonstrating the stomach and the portal sinus of the liver. The visceral situs should also be evaluated.

This is done by demonstrating the relative location of the stomach, hepatic vessels, abdominal aorta and inferior vena cava (**Figure 4**).

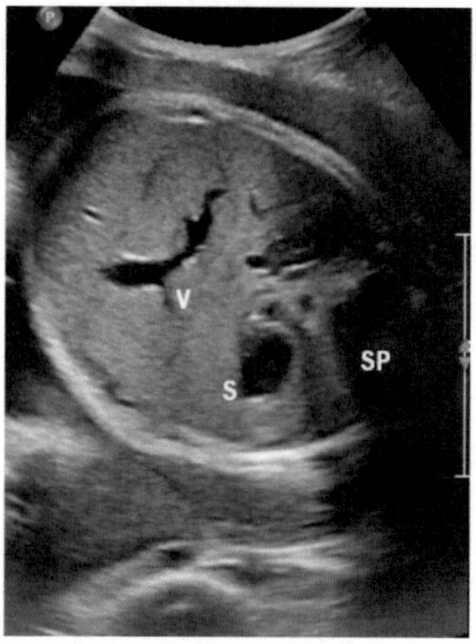

Figure 4.
Obstetric ultrasound showing the fetal abdomen. Fetal abdomen: The stomach (S) and intrahepatic portion of the umbilical vein (V) are demonstrated. The spine (SP) is seen posteriorly.

A case series of gastrointestinal abnormalities in fetuses with echogenic bowel detected during the antenatal period revealed that prenatal diagnosis of bowel abnormalities is challenging owing to the varying appearance of the bowel throughout pregnancy [26].

A related study showed that the prenatal ultrasound scan is unreliable in the detection or exclusion of fetal gastrointestinal malformations (GIM). Therefore clinicians involved in prenatal sonography or counseling should exercise caution in making such diagnoses. In this study, there were 220 confirmed cases of GIM, of which only 35 (16%) had been correctly identified prenatally. However, prenatal ultrasound was quite reliable in the detection of duodenal obstruction with 55% confirmed cases identified prenatally [27].

2.6 Kidneys and urinary tract

Detection of congenital urinary system anomalies is an important aspect of the prenatal ultrasound examination. Prenatal diagnosis of urinary tract abnormalities known to precipitate neonatal urosepsis and sequel such as renal scarring has made it possible to commence early intervention. A complete workup of the infants can be initiated early and before life-threatening complications occur.

The kidneys are visualized on sonography from as early as nine weeks of gestation and in all cases from twelve weeks. Echogenicity is high at nine weeks but reduces with advancing gestational age.

In a longitudinal scan, the kidneys are seen as elliptical structures while on axial sonograms, they are seen as rounded structures on either side of the spine. At 20 weeks, they show a hyperechoic capsule and the cortical area is slightly more echogenic than the medulla. Fat tissue normally accumulates around the kidneys as gestation progresses which enhances the borders of the kidneys in contrast with other organs. Normal ureters are rarely visualized in the absence of distal obstruction or reflux. The fetal bladder can be seen from the first trimester in more than 90% of subjects by 13 weeks (**Figure 5**).

A retrospective review of 56 children with urinary tract abnormalities detected by prenatal ultrasound revealed that more than half of the abnormalities were isolated hydronephrosis or multicystic dysplasia of the kidney [28].

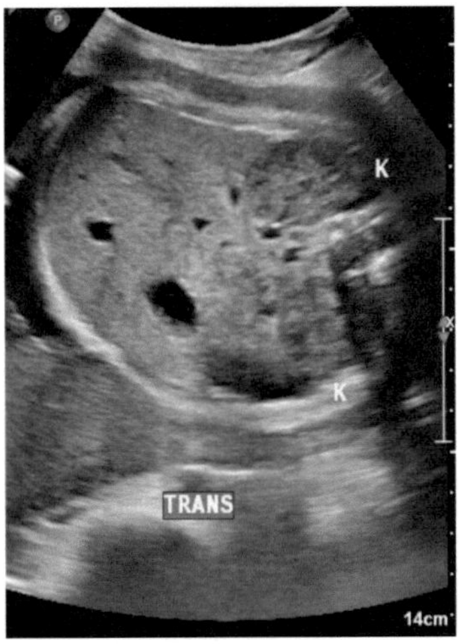

Figure 5.
Obstetric ultrasound showing fetal kidneys. Fetal abdomen at the level of the kidneys: Both kidneys (K) are seen on either side of the spine in this transverse sonogram.

The most frequent causes of hydronephrosis in the antenatal period are uretero-pelvic junction (UPJ) obstruction, ectopic ureterocele, and posterior urethral valves (PUV). Renal pelvis of more than 10 mm in anteroposterior diameter or more than half of the anteroposterior diameter of the kidney in transverse section are conclusive evidence of significant hydronephrosis.

2.7 Skeleton

Detection of fetal anomalies is satisfactory for most organ systems but remains poor for cardiac, skeletal, and craniofacial anomalies. In a study to assess the accuracy of the prenatal diagnosis of skeletal dysplasias by Barbara V. Parilla et al., the antenatal diagnosis was correct in 20 (65%) of 31 cases [29]. This suggests that precise antenatal diagnosis of skeletal dysplasia is challenging. However, the antenatal prediction of lethality was highly accurate.

In general, skeletal dysplasias are uncommon. They affect 1 in every 4,000–5,000 births, even though the incidence may be higher since the features may not be apparent until early childhood, at what time short stature, joint abnormalities or other complications become apparent.

Skeletal dysplasias comprise a heterogeneous group of disorders of skeletal growth that result in bones of abnormal size and shape.

Normally, all long bones are consistently seen from 11 weeks and the limbs move about readily at this gestation.

At the 18–23 week scan, the 3 segments of each limb should be visualized. It is nevertheless only necessary to measure the length of one femur. The relationship of the leg and foot should also be evaluated to rule out club foot.

US findings that are highly associated with the presence of a generalized skeletal dysplasia include shortening of extremity bones, fractures, bowing of long bones, demineralization, and a small thorax. A ratio of femur length to foot length of less than 0.9 and femur length–abdominal circumference ratio of less than 0.16 suggest a skeletal dysplasia.

3. Conclusion

Antenatal ultrasound can allow for early detection of fetal anomalies and therefore early intervention as well as appropriate management of the pregnancy.

Author details

Callen Kwamboka Onyambu[1]* and Norah Mukiri Tharamba[2]

1 Department of Diagnostic Imaging and Radiation Medicine, University of Nairobi, Nairobi, Kenya

2 Mathari Teaching and Referral Hospital, Nairobi, Kenya

*Address all correspondence to: callen.onyambu@uonbi.ac.ke

References

[1] R.M. S, D.I. S. Congenital malformations prevalent among Egyptian children and associated risk factors. Egyptian Journal of Medical Human Genetics. 2011.

[2] Samina Shamim, Nadeem Chohan SQ. Pattern of congenital malformations and their neonatal outcome. J Surg Pakistan Int. 2010;15(1):34-37.

[3] Alia N, Ahmed I, Mahais AH, Perveen N. Original Article CONGENITAL ANOMALIES : PREVALENCE OF CONGENITAL ABNORMALITIES IN 2 ND TRIMESTER OF PREGNANCY IN MADINA TEACHING HOSPITAL , FAISALABAD ON GRAY SCALE ULTRASOUND. J Univ Med Dent Coll. 2010;1(1):23-28.

[4] BI S, MS A-H, RA A, AA AS. Antenatal diagnosis, prevalence and outcome of major congenital anomalies in Saudi Arabia: a hospital-based study. Ann Saudi Med. 2008;

[5] Taboo ZA-A. Prevalence and Risk Factors for Congenital Anomalies in Mosul City. Iraqi Postgrad Med J. 2010;11(4).

[6] Barišić I, Group EW. EUROCAT – EPIDEMIOLOGICAL SURVEILLANCE OF CONGENITAL ANOMALIES IN EUROPE. Slov Med J [Internet]. 2018 Feb 14;78(0 SE-Review). Available from: https://vestnik.szd.si/index.php/ZdravVest/article/view/2760

[7] Improved National Prevalence Estimates for 18 Selected Major Birth Defects--United States, 1999-2001. JAMA J Am Med Assoc. 2006;

[8] Arjun Singh RKG. Pattern of Congenital Anomalies in Newborn: A Hospital Based Prospective Study. JK Sci. 2009;11(1):34-36.

[9] Magak P, King CH, Ireri E, Kadzo H, Ouma JH, Muchiri EM. High prevalence of ectopic kidney in Coast Province, Kenya. Trop Med Int Heal. 2004;

[10] Mashhadi Abdolahi H, Kargar Maher MH, Afsharnia F, Dastgiri S. Prevalence of Congenital Anomalies: A Community-Based Study in the Northwest of Iran. Neville H, Rice H, Tokiwa K, editors. ISRN Pediatr [Internet]. 2014;2014:920940. Available from: https://doi.org/10.1155/2014/920940

[11] Padma S, Ramakrishna D, Jijiya Bai P, Ramana P V. Pattern of distribution of congenital anomalies in stillborn: A hospital based prospective study. Int J Pharma Bio Sci. 2011;

[12] Ekwere EO, Mcneil R, Agim B, Jeminiwa B, Oni O, Pam S. A RETROSPECTIVE STUDY OF CONGENITAL ANOMALIES PRESENTED AT TERTIARY HEALTH FACILITIES IN JOS , NIGERIA. JPCS. 2011;

[13] Delport SD, Christianson AL, Van den Berg HJS, Wolmarans L, Gericke GS. Congenital anomalies in black South African liveborn neonates at an urban academic hospital. South African Med J. 1995;

[14] Onyambu CK, Tharamba NM. Screening for congenital fetal anomalies in low risk pregnancy: The Kenyatta National Hospital experience. BMC Pregnancy Childbirth. 2018;18(1).

[15] Parker A, Downs J, Kumar A, Shergill N, Jairaman, Jones AY-M, et al. Congenital anomalies fact sheet N 370. Pediatric Physical Therapy. 2014.

[16] Mashuda F, Zuechner A, Chalya PL, Kidenya BR, Manyama M. Pattern and factors associated with congenital anomalies among young infants

admitted at Bugando medical centre, Mwanza, Tanzania. BMC Res Notes. 2014;

[17] Martinez-Frías ML, Bermejo E, Rodríguez-Pinilla E, Frías JL. Congenital anomalies in the offspring of mothers with a bicornuate uterus. Pediatrics. 1998;

[18] Munim S, Nadeem S, Ali Khuwaja N. The accuracy of ultrasound in the diagnosis of congenital abnormalities. J Pak Med Assoc. 2006;

[19] Todros T, Capuzzo E, Gaglioti P. Prenatal diagnosis of congenital anomalies. Images Paediatr Cardiol [Internet]. 2001 Apr;3(2):3-18. Available from: https://pubmed.ncbi.nlm.nih.gov/22368596

[20] Johnson SP, Sebire NJ, Snijders RJM, Tunkel S, Nicolaides KH. Ultrasound screening for anencephaly at 10-14 weeks of gestation. Ultrasound Obstet Gynecol. 1997;

[21] Salomon LJ, Alfirevic Z, Berghella V, Bilardo C, Hernandez-Andrade E, Johnsen SL, et al. Practice guidelines for performance of the routine mid-trimester fetal ultrasound scan. Ultrasound Obstet Gynecol. 2011;

[22] Nicolaides KH, Azar G, Byrne D, Mansur C, Marks K. Fetal nuchal translucency: Ultrasound screening for chromosomal defects in first trimester of pregnancy. Br Med J. 1992;

[23] Benacerraf BR, Barss VA, Laboda LA. A sonographic sign for the detection in the second trimester of the fetus with Down's syndrome. Am J Obstet Gynecol. 1985;

[24] Ameh EA, Dogo PM, Nmadu PT. Emergency neonatal surgery in a developing country. Pediatr Surg Int. 2001;

[25] Abdur-Rahman L, Abdulrasheed N, Adeniran J. Challenges and outcomes of management of anterior abdominal wall defects in a Nigerian tertiary hospital. African J Paediatr Surg. 2011;

[26] Corteville JE, Gray DL, Langer JC. Bowel abnormalities in the fetus - Correlation of prenatal ultrasonographic findings with outcome. Am J Obstet Gynecol. 1996;

[27] Phelps S, Fisher R, Partington A, Dykes E. Prenatal ultrasound diagnosis of gastrointestinal malformations. In: Journal of Pediatric Surgery. 1997.

[28] Gloor JM, Ogburn PL, Breckle RJ, Morgenstern BZ, Milliner DS. Urinary Tract Anomalies Detected by Prenatal Ultrasound Examination at Mayo Clinic Rochester. Mayo Clin Proc. 1995;

[29] Parilla B V., Leeth EA, Kambich MP, Chilis P, MacGregor SN. Antenatal detection of skeletal dysplasias. J Ultrasound Med. 2003;

Chapter 10

Effect of Community-Based Intervention (Pregnant Women's Conference) on Institutional Delivery in Ethiopia

Melash Belachew Asresie and Gizachew Worku Dagnew

Abstract

Institutional delivery is the foundation for diminishing maternal mortality. Evidence showed that community-based behavioral change interventions are increasing institutional delivery in developing countries. By understanding this, the government of Ethiopia launched a community-based intervention called "pregnant women's conferences" to improve institutional delivery. This study was conducted to assess its effectiveness on institutional delivery among 871 women who gave birth within the last 12 months (435: pregnant women's conference attendants and 436: pregnant women's conference non-attendants) in 2017. It was a community-based comparative cross-sectional study and participants were selected using a multi-stage-simple random sampling technique. A structured interviewer-administered questionnaire was used for data collection. The result showed that institutional delivery among women who attended pregnant women's conferences was 54.3% (95%CI: 49.9–59.1), higher compared with 39.9% (95%CI: 35.3%- 44.7%) of women who did not attend the conference. Likewise, the level of well-preparedness for birth was higher among women who attended the conference (P = 38.9%, 95%CI: 33.8–43.7), compared with their counterparts (P = 25.7%, 95% CI: 22.2–29.4). Similarly, women's knowledge of obstetric danger signs was higher among women who attended the conference. Therefore, encouraging pregnant women to attend the conference should be strengthened.

Keywords: Pregnant women's conference, effect, pregnant, institutional delivery, Northwest, Ethiopia

1. Introduction

Birth assisted with skilled personnel is the foundation for reducing maternal Mortality. However, it is low in low and middle-income countries [1, 2]. Behavioral changing community-based interventions are globally recommended to increase institutional delivery by increasing obstetric danger signs and birth preparedness knowledge among women and the community [3, 4]. Low and middle-income countries have recently worked on behavior change interventions and mobilization of the community to increase institutional delivery and other maternal service utilization [5–7].

IntechOpen

To improve institutional delivery the public authority of Ethiopia has strived by introducing innovative practices like community participation such as the establishment of health development army at the village level, the adaptation of cultural practices at the health facility level such as preparation of "maternal waiting home", making the service free of charge and provision of charge-free transport service for pregnant women during labor and delivery. In this manner, acquires incredible changes in the use of maternal and childcare [8–11], however, still lagging behind the target. To overcome this challenge, the Ethiopian minister of health also launched recently a community-based intervention called "pregnant women's conference" (PWC) to enhance obstetric danger sign awareness and institutional skilled maternal health service utilization. The goal of PWC is to increase skilled maternal health care service, by reducing two delays (delay in deciding to seek care and delay to reach a health facility) through enhancing obstetric danger signs knowledge that may occur during pregnancy, childbirth, and postpartum period and inspire the women to prepare to childbirth and against the occurrence of any obstetric complication ahead of time.

The assigned Nurse/Midwifery provides education about Obstetric danger signs, antenatal care, institutional delivery, postnatal care, child care, child feeding, and immunizations. Each woman is expected to attend at least three conferences during each pregnancy. The service is delivering at their kebele level/the smallest administrative in Ethiopia/monthly and coordinated by community health workers called health Extention workers. As far as the authors are aware no study evaluated PWC intervention effectiveness on institutional delivery. Hence, this study was tried to evaluate the effect of PWC on institutional delivery by compared the prevalence of institutional delivery among women who attended PWC and women who did not attend the PWC during their last pregnancy in rural Northwest, Ethiopia.

2. Main body

2.1 Material and methods

2.1.1 Study area and period

The study was conducted in rural Libo Kemkem District Northwest Ethiopia from February 15 to March 26, 2017. It is 645 km away from Addis Ababa's capital city of Ethiopia. The district has 29 rural Kebeles & 5 urban Kebeles [12].

2.1.2 Study design, study population, and sample size

A comparative community-based cross-sectional study was carried out in women who gave birth within the last 12 months before the survey. For each group, the sample size was calculated using the two-sample comparisons of proportion formula using Epi-Info V.7, by considering the following assumptions: confidence level 95%, power 80, and the prevalence of institutional delivery in the intervention and the controlled group was 56% and 36%, respectively from the Burkina Faso study, as there is no similar study done in the study area [11]. Adding of 5% non-response rate and multiplied by 2 since we used the multistage sampling technique, the final minimum sample size calculated for each group was 450.

2.1.3 Sampling technique, data collection tool, process, and analysis

We used a multistage sampling technique to select 450 women for each group and each selected kebele. The first Seven rural kebele were selected using the lottery method of simple random sampling technique. Then women who gave birth in the last year prior to the survey at each selected kebele were grouped into two: pregnant women conference "attendants" and "non-attendants" using their family matrix book found from health post. After proportional allocation was done for each kebele computer generating simple random sampling technique was used to select study participants. A structured and pre-tested interviewer-administered questionnaire was used for data collection. The data was collected by trained data collectors using the local language Amharic. The tool was first developed in the English language then translated to the Amharic language. The collected data were coded and entered into EPI-Info version 7 and export to SPSS version 23 for analysis. Both descriptive and regression analyses were performed using binary logistic regression model. In the bivariate analysis variables with a P-value ≤ 0.20 were kept in the multivariable analysis to control the effect of confounders. Before doing independent logistic regression analysis for PWC attendants and non-attendants, a significant difference between the two groups was confirmed. Chi-square testing was done to see if there was a difference in institutional delivery utilization between the two groups (PWC attendants VS non-attendants) and a statistically significant difference was observed between the two groups (x^2 = 17.98, df = 1, p = <0.001), suggesting separate analysis. Odds ratios (AOR) with their 95% CI was calculated to measure the strength of association, and P-value ≤ 0.05 was considered as statistically significant.

2.2 Results

2.2.1 Socio-demographic and other characteristics of the respondents

About 96.7% of questionnaires distributed for PWC attendants and 96.9% of questionnaires distributed for PWC non-attendants were filled and analyzed. The mean age of women who attended the conference and did not attend the conference was 30.9 ± 5.5 years and 31.6 ± 5.1 years, respectively. Three-fourth (75.8%) of women who attended PWC and 60.9% of women who did not attend the PWC their age was 25–34 years. Above half (56.8%) and 45% of women who attended PWC and did not attend PWC were living with in1 hr. of walking from the nearest health facility. The majority of women, 92.2% of women who attended the PWC and 78.0% of women who did not attend the PWC were had at least one ANC visit during their last pregnancy. Three-fourth (72.6%) of women who attended the PWC and 55% of women who did not attend the PWC had discussed the place of delivery. Half of the women who attended the PWC and 56.4% of women who did not attend the PWC gave birth at a health institution before the index birth. About 1.4% of women who attended PWC and 3.4% of women who did not attend the PWC had experienced stillbirth (**Table 1**).

2.2.2 Awareness of obstetric danger signs

Each woman was asked to mention the key danger signs that can happen during pregnancy, childbirth, and the postpartum period. Accordingly, about 99.8% and 95.4% of women who attended and did not attend the PWC were committed to mention at least one obstetric key danger sign that may occur during pregnancy, childbirth, or postpartum periods. About 62% and 40% of women who attended and did not attend the PWC were mentioned severe vaginal bleeding as a dangerous sign during pregnancy, respectively (**Table 2**).

2.2.3 Obstetric danger signs knowledge

In this study, a mother was considered as *knowledgeable on pregnancy danger signs* if she mentioned at least two of the three key danger signs (severe vaginal bleeding,

Variable	Variable Categories	PWC non-attendants (n = 436)	PWC attendants (n = 435)
		n (%)	n (%)
Age of women (years)	19–24	62(14.2)	41(9.4)
	25–34	252(75.8)	265(60.9)
	> = 35	122(28)	129(29.7)
Educational status	Unable to read and write	379(86.9)	401(92.2)
	Can read and write	0(0.0)	2(0.5)
	Grade 1–8	51(11.7)	32(7.4)
	Secondary and above	6(1.4)	0(0.0)
Occupation	Housewife	417(95.6)	430(98.9)
	Farmer	11(2.5)	5(1.1)
	Governmental employee	8(1.8)	0(0.0)
Marital status	Divorce	9(2.1)	5(1.1)
	Widowed	2(0.5)	1(0.2)
	Married	425(97.5)	429(98.6)
Family size	≤4	113(25.9)	125(28.7)
	> = 5	323(74.1)	310(71.3)
Husbands' education	Unable to read and write	271(67.8)	263(61.3)
	Can read and write	102(24.0)	118(27.5)
	Grade 1–8	35(8.24)	40(9.3)
	Secondary and above	17(4)	8(1.9)
Husbands' Occupation	Farmer	407(95.8)	419(95.6)
	Governmental employee	18(4.24)	10(2.3)

Table 1.
Socio-demographic characteristics of women who gave birth in the last 12 months, in the context of attending PWC, Northwest Ethiopia, 2017.

Variables	Categories	PWC non-attendants' n (%)	PWC attendants' n (%)
Danger signs			
During pregnancy	Severe vaginal bleeding	176 (40.4)	269 (61.8)
	Swollen of hands and face	151 (34.6)	214 (49.2)
	Blurred vision	92 (21.1)	110 (25.3)
During childbirth	Sever vaginal bleeding	118 (27.1)	182 (41.8)
	Prolonged labor (>12 hrs)	129 (29.6)	174 (40)
	Convulsion	35 (8.0)	68 (15.6)
	Retained placenta	287 (67.4)	309 (71.2)
During postpartum	Severe Vaginal bleeding	182 (42.7)	267 (61.5)
	Foul-smelling vaginal discharge	79 (18.5)	166 (38.2)
	High fever	11 (2.6)	53 (12.2)

Table 2.
Awareness of obstetric danger signs among women who gave birth in the last 12 months, in the context of attending PWC, Northwest Ethiopia, 2017.

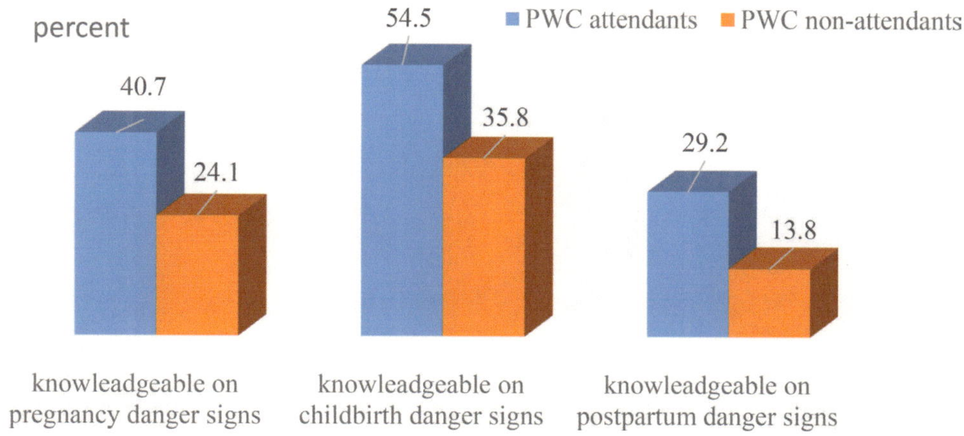

Figure 1.
Knowledge of obstetric danger signs among women who gave birth in the last 12 months, in the context of attending PWC, Northwest Ethiopia, 2017.

swollen hands/face, and blurred vision) that may occur during pregnancy, *knowledgeable on childbirth danger signs* if she mentioned at least two of the four key danger signs (severe vaginal bleeding, prolonged labor (>12 hours), convulsion, and placenta retained) may happen during labor, and *knowledgeable on postpartum danger signs* if she mentioned at least two of the three key danger signs (severe vaginal bleeding, foul-smelling vaginal discharge, and high fever) may happen during the postpartum period. According to this definition, about 41% and 24% of women who attended and did not attend PWC were knowledgeable (mentioned at least two danger signs) on pregnancy danger signs, respectively (**Figure 1**).

2.2.4 Birth and its complication readiness practice during their last pregnancy

All women were asked what they prepared before the onset of labor during their last pregnancy. Almost three-fourth (73.3%) of women who attended the PWC and half (54.4%) of women who did not attend the PWC, reported that they were planned health facilities for delivery. About 42% of PWC attendants and 29% of PWC non-attendants were saved money for an emergency before the onset of labor (**Figure 2**).

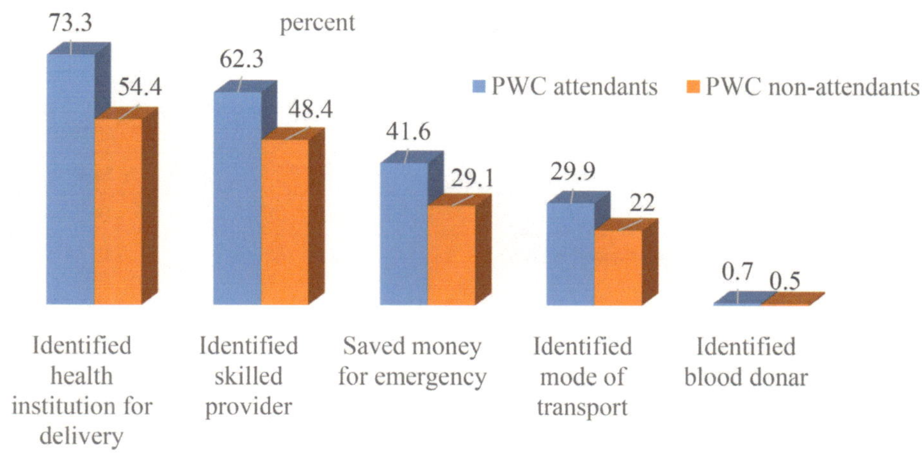

Figure 2.
Birth preparedness and complication readiness practice among women who gave birth in the last 12 months, in the context of attending PWC, Northwest Ethiopia, 2017.

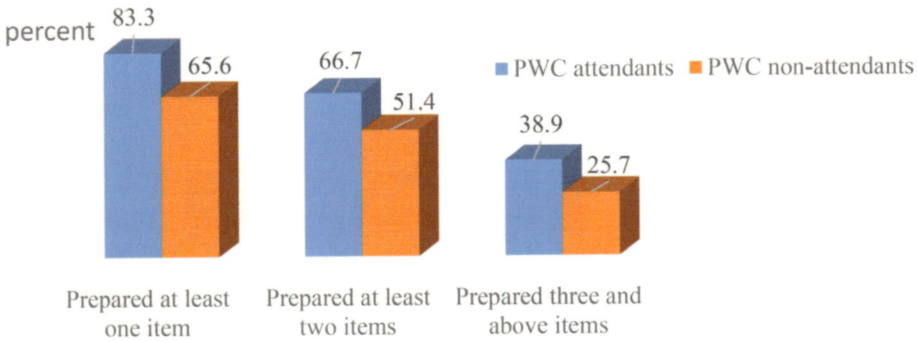

Figure 3.
Well-preparedness during their last pregnancy among women who gave birth in the last 12 month, in the context of attending PWC, Northwest Ethiopia, 2017.

2.2.5 Well-preparedness practice during their last pregnancy

A mother was considered as "*well-prepared for institutional delivery* "if she prepared at least three items from the four key items (identified the skilled provider, saved money, planned health facility for delivery, and identified the mode of transportation) during her last pregnancy before the onset of labor. According, to the total, 38.9% of women who attended the PWC (95%CI: 33.8-43.7), and 25.7% of women who didn't attend the PWC (95% CI: 22.2-29.4) were "well-prepared" for birth and its complication during their last pregnancy before the onset of labor (**Figure 3**).

2.2.6 Place of planned for delivery and delivery

Every woman was expected to choose a health institution for delivery, however, about 73.3% of PWC attendants and 54.4% of PWC non-attendant women only were planned health institutions to birth. Close attention from their families or relatives was the most frequently mentioned reason why they preferred home for birth (**Table 3**).

Variables	PWC non-attendants n1 (%)	PWC attendants n2 (%)
A planned place for the birth		
health institution	237(54.4)	319(73.3)
home	199(45.6)	116(26.7)
Why planned home for delivery (n1 = 199, n2 = 116)		
They feel more comfortable giving birth at home	121(60.8)	65 (56.0)
Close attention from their families and relatives	98(49.2)	54 (46.6)
Their usual practice	39(19.6)	19 (16.4)
They did not like the service provided in health facilities	29(14.6)	13 (11.2)
They had a bad experience giving birth at a health facility	4 (2.0)	2(1.7)
Their family's preference	16(8.0)	3(2.6)
The unwelcoming approach of health care workers	5 (2.5)	2(1.7)

Table 3.
The planned place for delivery and reasons to plan among women who gave birth in the last 12 months, in the context of attending PWC, Northwest Ethiopia, 2017.

Variables	PWC non-attendants n (%)	PWC attendants n (%)
Place of delivery		
At the health center	139(31.9)	206(47.4)
At hospital	35(8.0)	30(6.9)
Home	262(60.1)	199(45.7)
Why delivered at home after planned health institution (n1 = 88,n2 = 81)		
Labor was urgent to reach a health facility	28(31.8)	32(39.5)
Labor was coming at night and wait till dawn	32 (36.4)	47(58.0)
Lack of transport	25(28.4)	18(22.2)
Lack of person look after home and care children	15(17.0)	18(22.1)
Family members prefer to deliver at home	17(19.3)	8(9.9)
The birth outcome of the current delivery		
Alive	428(98.2)	432(99.3)
Stillbirth	8(1.8)	3(0.7)
Postnatal care in the current delivery		
At least 1 visit	141(32.3)	229(52.6)
At least 2 visits	59(13.5)	97(22.3)
3 and above visits	10(2.3)	23(5.3)
No visit	295(67.7)	206(47.4)

Table 4.
Institutional delivery among women who gave birth in the last 12 months, in the context of attending PWC, Northwest Ethiopia, 2017.

2.2.7 Institutional delivery

Overall institutional delivery was 47.1%(95%CI:43.4–50.9). It was 54.3% (95%CI: 49.9–59.1) among women who attended the PWC and 39.9% (95%CI: 35.3%-44.7%) among women who did not attend the PWC. Regarding postnatal follow up visits, only 22.3% of PWC attendants and 13.5% of PWC non-attendant were had two or more visits during the index birth (**Table 4**).

2.2.8 Factors associated with institutional delivery

Both bivariate and multivariable analyses were performed. As **Table 5** showed that during multivariable analysis variables such as knowledge on childbirth and postpartum danger signs, traveling time to reach the nearest health facility, well prepared for birth and its complication, and discussion with partners/families about the place of birth were significantly associated with institutional delivery in women who attended the PWC. Whereas among women who did not attend the conference knowledge on pregnancy danger signs, traveling time to reach the nearest health facility, and well prepared for birth and its complication were significantly associated with institutional delivery. Among women who attended the PWC those who were knowledgeable on childbirth danger signs were 1.7 times more likely to deliver at health institutions compared to women who were not knowledgeable on childbirth danger signs (AOR = 1.7, 95%CI: 1.2, 2.8).

Variables	PWC attendants				PWC non-attendants			
	I. delivery		COR	AOR	I. delivery		COR	AOR
	Yes	No			Yes	No		
Travel time to a nearby health facility								
<=1 hour on foot	181	66	6.6(4.3,10.1)	4.4(2.4,8.1) *	131	65	9.2(5.9,14.4)	7.8(4.4,13.7*)
>1 hour on foot	55	133	1	1	43	65	1	1
Discussed with partner/family about the place of birth								
No	15	104	1	1	46	149	1	
Yes	221	95	16.1(8.9,29.0)	7.7(3.6,16.4) *	128	113	3.7(2.4,5.6)	======
Knowledge of at least two danger signs of pregnancy								
No	92	166	1		89	242	1	1
Yes	144	33	7.9(5.0,12.4)	========	85	20	11.6(6.7,19.9)	3.6(1.6,8.1) *
Knowledge of at least two danger signs of childbirth								
No	64	134	1	1	85	159	1	
Yes	172	65	5.5(3.7,8.4)	1.7(1.2,2.8) *	89	67	3.0(2.0,4.6)	======
Knowledge of at least two danger signs of postpartum								
No	113	195	1	1	115	261	1	
Yes	123	4	53.1(19.1,147.5)	14.0(4.6,40.0) *	59	1	133.9(18.3,978.3)	======
Well prepared								
No	77	189	1	1	88	236	1	1
Yes	159	10	39.0(19.5,77.9)	8.8(3.9,19.8) *	86	26	8.9(5.4,14.7)	3.3(1.6,7.0) *

*Key I. delivery=institutional delivery *=statically significant associated at p-value ≤ 0.05*

Table 5.
Factors associated with institutional delivery among women who gave birth in the last 12 months, in the context of attending PWC, Northwest Ethiopia, 2017.

Whereas, in women who did not attend PWC the Odds of institutional delivery among women who were knowledgeable on pregnancy danger signs were 3.6 times higher compared with their counterparts (AOR = 3.6, 95%CI: 1.6, 8.1) (**Table 5**).

2.3 Discussion

This study intended to assess the effectiveness of a community-based intervention called PWC on institutional delivery in the Northwest part of Ethiopia. Accordingly, institution delivery was higher among women who attended the PWC was 54.3% (95%CI: 49.9–59.1) compared to 39.9% (95%CI: 35.3%- 44.7%) in women who did not attend the PWC. Other previous studies supported this finding, Burkina Faso (56% VS 36%), Eritrea (46.8% VS 51.2), and Guatemala (54.7% VS 31.2%) [11–13], authors agreed that women who involved in the conference were informed about danger signs that may occur during delivery, which enable them to prefer health institution for delivery [14]. On the contrary of this finding, studies were done in Kenya (28% VS 37%), Bangladesh (10.5% VS 12.5%), and India (22.5% VS 21.8%) showed that the community-based interventions were not made difference on institutional delivery as compared to their counterpart [15, 16].

Similarly, knowledge of obstetric danger signs that may occur during pregnancy, labor, and postpartum was higher among women who attended the PWC compared to those women who did not attend the PWC. This finding was in line with the studies done in Eritrea, and Bangladesh [12, 16]. Conversely, this finding was contradicted with the studies done in Nepal and Bangladesh, which showed that obstetric danger signs knowledge of women who were involved in the intervention were similar or lower compared to women not participating in the interventions [17, 18].

About 39% of women who attended the PWC were well prepared for birth and its complication higher as compared to 28% of women who did not attend the PWC before the onset of labor, was supported with previous studies done in Burkina Faso, Eretria, Nepal, and Tanzania the higher level of well-preparedness for birth and its complication was made among women who participated in the interventions [6, 12, 19, 20]. The explanation may be women who are involved in the intervention might be informed about obstetric danger signs and birth preparedness items which elicit them to be ready to give birth at a health institution.

The odds of institutional delivery among PWC attendant women who were knowledgeable about childbirth and postpartum danger signs were higher as compared to their counterparts. Then again, among PWC non-attendant women who were knowledgeable on pregnancy danger signs were more likely to institutional delivery compared to their counterparts. It was supported by the previous studies done in Ethiopia, Pakistan, and Tanzania [14, 21, 22]. The possible clarification may be realizing obstetric threat signs may impact women's perceptions about their susceptibility to and earnestness of the complications. This may motivate women to give birth at wellbeing offices [23].

The odds of institutional delivery among both groups of women who well-prepared for birth and its complication were higher as compared not prepared. The explanation may be women who were solid and steady for birth and its complexity may be proficient about obstetric danger signs that may happen before, during, and after birth; decidedly impact to delivery at a health facility.

Voyaging time from the closest health facility was essentially connected with institutional delivery in both women who joined in and did not go to the PWC. In both groups, women who lived within 1 h of strolling from the closest health facility were more likely to institutional delivery contrasted with their counterparts. This finding was in line with other previous studies [14, 23–25]. The explanation may be an absence of methods for transportation to wellbeing offices. Secondly, fear of financial expense for transport may be contrarily affected to choose institutional delivery.

The odds of institutional delivery among PWC attendant women who had a conversation with partners/families about the place of birth were higher as compared to women who did not discuss. This may empower women to have self-rule in the decision of birthplace jointly or self alone. Women with the highest level of autonomy are most likely to seek institutional delivery [21, 26–28]. Also, this may set out a better opportunity for families to include in orchestrating transport, set aside cash, and assist mothers to choose a place of delivery.

2.4 Limitation of this study

The two group participants (PWC attendants and non-attendants) live at the same resident/kebele, there might be information contamination between attendants and non-attendants.

2.5 Conclusion

The proportion of institutional delivery was higher among women who attended the conference. Similarly, women's knowledge of obstetric danger signs and preparation for birth and its complication were higher among women who attended the conference. Knowledge on childbirth and postpartum danger signs, discussed with their partners/families about the place of delivery were associated with institutional delivery in Pregnant women's conference attendants. Distance from the nearest health facility and well preparedness for birth and its complication were associated with institutional delivery in both groups. Besides, knowledge of pregnancy danger signs was associated with institutional delivery in pregnant women's conference non-attendants.

Therefore, strengthening women to attend pregnant women's conferences may improve institutional delivery by increasing women's obstetric danger signs and birth preparedness knowledge. Furthermore, encouraging women to discuss with their families about the place of delivery should be strengthened.

For researchers, the authors recommended doing a further follow-up cluster-based study by considering a non-selected zone (buffer zone) between intervention and control groups to prevent information contamination, thereby, understanding the net effect of the intervention in the institutional delivery.

Acknowledgements

We would like to express our gratitude to Bahir Dar University, Amhara regional health bureau, South Gondar Zone Health Office, LiboKmem district Health Office, data collectors and supervisors, Health Extention workers, and study participants for their contribution.

Competing interests

The authors declare that they have no competing interests.

Ethical approval and consent to participate

Ethical clearance was obtained from the IRB committee of Bahir Dar University. Permission letter also received from the region, zonal department, and district health office. Written consent was obtained from each study participant. To ensure confidentiality identification such as name was not recorded. The purpose of the study was explained to each participant.

Author details

Melash Belachew Asresie* and Gizachew Worku Dagnew
Department of Reproductive Health and Population Studies, School of Public Health, College of Medicine and Health Sciences, Bahir Dar University, Bahir Dar, Ethiopia

*Address all correspondence to: kalleab1@gmail.com

References

[1] Demographic, I.E., *Health Survey 2016: Key Indicators Report. Addis Ababa, Ethiopia, and Rockville, Maryland, USA.* CSA and ICF, 2016.

[2] Assefa, Y., et al., *Successes and challenges of the millennium development goals in Ethiopia: lessons for the sustainable development goals.* BMJ global health, 2017. **2**(2): p. e000318.

[3] Mbalinda, S.N., et al., *Does knowledge of danger signs of pregnancy predict birth preparedness? A critique of the evidence from women admitted with pregnancy complications.* Health research policy and systems, 2014. **12**(1): p. 60.

[4] Nawal, D. and S. Goli, *Birth preparedness and its effect on place of delivery and post-natal check-ups in Nepal.* PloS one, 2013. **8**(5): p. e60957.

[5] Skinner, J. and T. Rathavy, *Design and evaluation of a community participatory, birth preparedness project in Cambodia.* Midwifery, 2009. **25**(6): p. 738-743.

[6] Moran, A.C., et al., *Birth-preparedness for maternal health: findings from Koupéla district, Burkina Faso.* Journal of health, population, and nutrition, 2006. **24**(4): p. 489.

[7] Mushi, D., R. Mpembeni, and A. Jahn, *Effectiveness of community-based safe motherhood promoters in improving the utilization of obstetric care. The case of Mtwara Rural District in Tanzania.* BMC pregnancy and childbirth, 2010. **10**(1): p. 14.

[8] Medhanyie, A., et al., *The role of health extension workers in improving utilization of maternal health services in rural areas in Ethiopia: a cross-sectional study.* BMC health services research, 2012. **12**(1): p. 352.

[9] Banteyerga, H., *Ethiopia's health extension program: improving health through community involvement.* MEDICC Review, 2011. **13**(3): p. 46-49.

[10] *LKDHOffice. Annual Report 2016/17, Amhar Region NW, Ethiopia.2017.*

[11] Brazier, E., et al., *Improving poor women's access to maternity care: Findings from a primary care intervention in Burkina Faso.* Social science & medicine, 2009. **69**(5): p. 682-690.

[12] Turan, J.M., M. Tesfagiorghis, and M.L. Polan, *Evaluation of a community intervention for the promotion of safe motherhood in Eritrea.* Journal of midwifery & women's health, 2011. **56**(1): p. 8-17.

[13] *Family Care International. Care–seeking during pregnancy, delivery and the postpartum period: A Study in Homabay and Migori Districts, Kenya. FCI; 2003.*

[14] Mpembeni, R.N., et al., *Use pattern of maternal health services and determinants of skilled care during delivery in Southern Tanzania: implications for achievement of MDG-5 targets.* BMC pregnancy and childbirth, 2007. **7**(1): p. 29.

[15] Baqui, A., et al., *Impact of an integrated nutrition and health program on neonatal mortality in rural northern India.* Bulletin of the World Health Organization, 2008. **86**: p. 796-804A.

[16] Hossain, J. and S. Ross, *The effect of addressing the demand for as well as the supply of emergency obstetric care in Dinajpur, Bangladesh.* International Journal of Gynecology & Obstetrics, 2006. **92**(3): p. 320-328.

[17] Sood, S., et al., *Measuring the effects of behavior change interventions in Nepal with population-based survey results.* 2004.

[18] Darmstadt, G.L., et al., *Evaluation of a cluster-randomized controlled trial of a package of community-based maternal*

and newborn interventions in Mirzapur, Bangladesh. PloS one, 2010. **5**(3): p. e9696.

[19] McPherson, R.A., et al., *Are birth-preparedness programs effective? Results from a field trial in Siraha district, Nepal.* Journal of health, population, and nutrition, 2006. **24**(4): p. 479.

[20] August, F., *Effect of Home-Based Life-Saving Skills education on knowledge of obstetric danger signs, birth preparedness, utilization of skilled care and male involvement: A Community-based intervention study in rural Tanzania*. 2016, Acta Universitatis Upsaliensis.

[21] Tura, G., *Safe delivery service utilization in Metekel zone, northwest Ethiopia.* Ethiopian Journal of Health Sciences, 2008. **18**(1).

[22] Agha, S. and T.W. Carton, *Determinants of institutional delivery in rural Jhang, Pakistan.* International journal for equity in health, 2011. **10**(1): p. 31.

[23] Alemi Kebede, K.H. and A.N. Teklehaymanot, *Factors associated with institutional delivery service utilization in Ethiopia.* International journal of women's health, 2016. **8**: p. 463.

[24] Yanagisawa, S., S. Oum, and S. Wakai, *Determinants of skilled birth attendance in rural Cambodia.* Tropical Medicine & International Health, 2006. **11**(2): p. 238-251.

[25] Stekelenburg, J., et al., *Waiting too long: low use of maternal health services in Kalabo, Zambia.* Tropical Medicine & International Health, 2004. **9**(3): p. 390-398.

[26] Fikre, A.A. and M. Demissie, *Prevalence of institutional delivery and associated factors in Dodota Woreda (district), Oromia regional state, Ethiopia.* Reproductive health, 2012. **9**(1): p. 33.

[27] Hagos, S., et al., *Utilization of institutional delivery service at Wukro and Butajera districts in the Northern and South Central Ethiopia.* BMC pregnancy and childbirth, 2014. **14**(1): p. 178.

[28] Asefa, A., et al., *Mismatch between antenatal care attendance and institutional delivery in south Ethiopia: A multilevel analysis.* BMJ Open, 2019. **9**(3): p. e024783.

Chapter 11

Domestic Violence in Pregnant Women and Their Types. Case Study in Bali, Indonesia

Ni Komang Yuni Rahyani, Ni Made Dwi Mahayati, Made Widhi Gunapria Darmapatni and Ni Wayan Armini

Abstract

The island of Bali, as part of the Republic of Indonesia, is predominantly Hindu and generally follows a patrilineal kinship system. There is a link between the patrilineal kinship system and incidents of violence against women. The purpose of this paper is to describe the incidence of domestic violence /DV that has been experienced by pregnant women in the last 12 months in Bali. The study design was a mixed method, namely quantitative-qualitative. The research samples were pregnant women in the third trimester in the Pedungan Traditional Village area in Denpasar City (31 people) and the Nongan Traditional Village in Karangasem Regency (33 people). Data collection was carried out in 2015 from June to August. Forms of domestic violence incidents experienced by pregnant women in the last 12 months were more pregnant women in Nongan Village experiencing sexual abuse (3 people / 9.09% vs. 2 people / 6.45%)), economic abuse incidents (8 people / 24.24% vs. 2 people / 6.45%) compared to pregnant women in Pedungan Village. History of DV in the form of physical violence, social violence and emotional violence. The negative impact felt by pregnant women who are victims of DV, especially psychosomatic complaints, even to the point where they intend to suicide, delayed in doing antenatal care and miscarriage. It is necessary to improve the role and competence of midwives in early detection of DV in pregnant women who have their antenatal care at a health facility and cross-sector cooperation.

Keywords: Domestic violence, pregnant women, patrilineal, sexual abuse, economic abuse

1. Introduction

Indonesia is an archipelago with 17,550 islands. Indonesia has a variety of different cultures from one island to another. The majority of religions embraced by people in Indonesia is Islam. In Islam there are some controversial issues related to gender relations, including the question of the origin of women's creation, the concept of inheritance, witnessing, polygamy, reproductive rights, divorce rights, and the public role of women. If at a glance the text of the verses relating to the problem suggests an imbalance or injustice towards women [1].

According to data from the National Committee for the Protection of Women and Children in Indonesia in 2019, there were 431,471 cases of violence against women.

This figure is an increase of 693% from 2008 which was only 54,425 cases. This data is the tip of the iceberg, because there are still many unknown events. In 2019, 66 cases of violence against women, especially domestic violence, 41 cases of violence occurred in the workplace, 39 cases of violence occurred in public spaces, 14 cases of violence against women, 11 cases of violence in media facilities, and 6 cases of violence were reported experienced by migrant workers. The most common form of violence against women was sexual violence committed by friends or neighbors of victims.

The Bali Island is one of the provinces in Indonesia which has been known to have very high artistic and cultural appeal. The majority of the population on the island of Bali is Hindu. Data based from the central statistics agency of Bali Province in 2014 reported that amount 3,729,893 out of 4,365,107 people on the island of Bali are Hindus. The controlling holder of Balinese life is the customary village or *Desa Adat*, so that almost all individual activities are full of customary sequences. "Adat" also means regulations, laws, moral standards that guide all Balinese. Balinese people are said to have succeeded in maintaining cultural values because of the strong religious traditions. The role of members of traditional villages and their officials in Bali has a very big role in the social sector, including health. According to customary law, the position of Balinese women is under men or sub-ordinations [2]. The consequences is the incidence of domestic violence (DV) in the scope of customary villages in Bali tends to be influenced by the pattern of family relationships, especially husband-wife, in which men or husbands perceive women or wives as property rights.

Problems that are very closely related to gender issues include violence against women, and this condition occurs across countries, cultures and religions. Violence against women can occur throughout a woman's life and has a negative impact on women's health in the future. Domestic violence is the most common part of violence against women. In fact, there are still many women who do not realize that domestic violence must end. This is due to ignorance, culture, religious values, beliefs and the lack of optimal laws and regulations regarding the eradication of violence against women. The problem of domestic violence is considered as the domestic domain, not the public domain [3, 4].

Incidence of violence against women especially among pregnant women triggers a high risk of miscarriage, unsafe abortion, premature labor, and fetal distress, pregnant women who are late in checking their pregnancies, low nutritional status, contracting sexually transmitted diseases (STDs), unwanted pregnancies, as well as other infections [5–8]. There is a relationship between violence against women and the birth of low birth weight babies (LBW) especially in developing countries. Approximately 16% of all maternal mortality in India during pregnancy are a result of DV [9, 10].

Domestic violence is influenced by several factors that are interrelated with one another, as described in the "ecological framework. In the context of this research, the term used is domestic violence (DV) which can also be referred to as domestic violence (DV) [9]. The definition of gender-based violence according to the United Nations (1993), when it ratified the Declaration on the Elimination of Violence against Women, is:

"Gender-based violence includes actions or attempts to dominate men against women, including actions that can injure physically, mentally, socially, sexually and various forms of action that degrading the dignity of women" [11].

"The term "violence against women" can occur in both the private and public sphere and is experienced throughout the life cycle of women. Violence can take the form of beatings or hurting physically, emotionally, sexually and even socially" [12]. There is a term intimate partner violence (IPV) which is another form of violence against women. Acts of violence are generally carried out by their closest people or partners. The resulting impact is also very large on the health and well-being of women. The point is that women must submit to men and follow the rules they make [13].

The terminology of gender-based violence or violence against women that is commonly used is a model of violence in the domestic sphere. Domestic violence acts in the domestic sphere or household is a hidden stigma [14]. Domestic violence (DV) is a threat or abuses physically, psychologically and emotionally to women by other people who have the power to suppress and even force victims/women in the household [7]. Typical interpreters are people who are known or close to the victim, namely: husband, girlfriend, intimate partner, siblings, in-laws, in-laws, friends and other people. There are different patterns regarding perpetrators and victims of violence based on gender. More violence experienced by men is obtained from the social or public environment, while violence against women is carried out by social relations or people who are closely related to women [9].

2. Methods

This research was a mixed method (quantitative-qualitative) which was conducted from June to August 2015. The samples involved were pregnant women in the third trimester in the Pedungan Traditional Village area in Denpasar City (31 people) and in Nongan Village in Karangasem Regency (33 people). The location selection was based on the consideration that the two areas represented the living conditions of the people in Traditional Villages in urban areas and in rural areas in Bali. Traditional Village is the foundation of community life in Bali. The instruments used were self-reported questionnaires, in-depth interview guides and observation sheets. The data collector recorded the results of the interview using a recorder which was then translated into notes.

Quantitative data analysis used univariate test in the form of proportions, bivariate analysis with Chi-square test. Qualitative analysis with content analysis. Data on the history of violence by husbands were obtained from husbands through in-depth interviews. Due to confidentiality and safety reasons from the respondent, the researchers explored information about the history of DV incidents experienced by women without their husbands. Likewise, when researchers asked for information about acts of violence against women that had been committed by husbands in the last 12 months. Researchers also provided some equipment in the form of tissues and candy when collecting data because the questions were very sensitive and caused respondents to recall painful events they had experienced. The husbands of pregnant women were also included in this study. Questions to husbands were related to their previous experience in the last 12 months, whether or not they had committed acts of violence against their wives and what was the reason.

3. Results and discussion

3.1 Domestic violence form

There are several forms of violence against women according to the life cycle according to the World Health Organization (WHO), namely: pre-birth, infancy, girlhood, adolescence and adulthood, and elderly. The form of violence in the prebirth phase is in the form of abortion due to gender selection and due to blows and kicks on the mother's stomach. Child marriage, female genital mutilation, physical, sexual and psychological abuse, incest, child prostitution and pornography is a form of violence that most often occurs in girlhood phases. Dating violence and courtship violence (e.g. rape or forced sex with threats), forced sex work due to economic pressure (e.g. marital rape, dowry abuse and murders), partner homicide, psychological abuse, abuse of women with disabilities, and forced pregnancy is a form of violence that most often occurs in adolescence and adulthood phases [15].

Based on data of National Commission on Violence Against Women of Indonesia (2020), recorded that the most reported area of violence cases is domestic violence (DV) or personal sphere. The percentage reached 69% of the total cases during January–May 2020. This was followed by violence in the community (30%) and state (1%). Women experience higher incidence of violence due to low education, economic dependence, parenting in families that accept violence and give boys special treatment. Studies estimate that, from country to country, between 20 and 50 per cent of women have experienced physical violence at the hands of an intimate partner or family member [16].

Forms or manifestations of violence against women include physical, emotional or psychological abuse, sexual, social and economic abuse [9, 15, 17–19]. According to Digest (2000), found that physical abuse such as slapping, beating, arm twisting, stabbing, strangling, burning, choking, kicking, threats with an object or weapon, and murder. It also includes traditional practices that harm women's reproductive health, such as genital mutilation and sexual abuse. Psychological abuse takes the form of threats that can cause deep trauma to the victim. Economic abuse includes actions such as not providing expenses or income to the wife/partner to pay for household needs, as well as costs for maternity care and access to health care facilities. Social abuse includes the perpetrator prevents the wife/woman from meeting or socializing with friends including relatives and other close family members. This includes blocking the use of means of communication/telephone [5, 8, 9, 15, 16, 18, 20, 21].

In general, the role and function of midwives in the community regarding early detection and management of women victims of DV is still very limited, especially in Indonesia. The results of a study conducted by the National Committee for Women in Indonesia (2019) obtained data from 2008 to 2019 there was an increase in the incidence of violence against women from 54,425 cases to 431,471 cases. The increase in cases is almost tenfold. The most reported form of violence against women was DV, amounting to 71% or as many as 9,637 cases. The highest reported forms of DV were physical violence (3,927 cases/41%), sexual violence (2,988 cases/31%), psychological violence (1,658 cases/17%) and economic violence (1,064 cases/11%). The province known for the highest domestic violence report until 2019 was West Java (2,738 cases), followed by Central Java Province (2,525 cases), Capital city of Jakarta (2,222 cases). Data from the Integrated Service Center for the Empowerment of Women and Children in Denpasar City (2019), it was found that there was an increase in the number of cases of domestic violence from 2014 to 2018 by more than 100%, from 4 cases to 47 cases. The cases of sexuality also reported increase from 4 cases to 16 cases or increased fourfold from 2014 to 2018. Unfortunately, the incidence of violence during pregnancy is not available data in a large scale. The results of a study in Bali (2015), found that as many as 1 in 4 pregnant women have been victims of violence by their husbands or partners in the last 12 months [18].

3.2 Pregnant woman and partner characteristic

There was a significant difference in the characteristics of the respondents according to the level of education of the mother and the husband's education. Gender inequality [22, 23], culture, norms, values, beliefs [8, 9], lower socioeconomic status [24] as a risk factor for domestic violence among pregnant women. Male partners who abuse alcohol or use drugs, are unemployed or intermittently employed, have less than a high-school education is the cause of the increase in violence against women [23, 25].

The ecological framework in violence against women includes: individual level have been a victim of violence in the family, for examples: become addicted to alcohol and illegal substances and parenting; relationship level (such as family, friends, intimate partners and peers may influence the risks of becoming a victim or perpetrator of violence); Community level (social relationships occur, such as schools, neighborhoods and workplaces, also influence violence); and societal level (influence whether violence is encouraged or inhibited. There is an understanding that acts of violence are considered as a natural thing for men to do against women to maintain economic stability, avoid social conflicts, and even perpetuate subordination. [3, 9, 19, 21, 23, 26–28] (**Table 1**).

3.3 The experience of domestic violence by partner or husband

It is known that globally, more than one third of women aged 15 to 64 have been victims of violence by an intimate partner or husband. This number is consistent with global figures on gender-based violence [29]. The condition of women in Bali, who are predominantly Hindu, has a marriage value in the form of "mesatya". "Mesatya" is a value about loyalty to their spouse or husband and the husband family to death. Or the same as the principle of getting married once in a lifetime. No matter how difficult the problems faced when married, it must remain obedient and obedient to her husband and family. One factor that triggers the DV is that the value or belief that women or wives are the property of their husbands, the husband has the right and is accepted if he treats his wife at will [2, 19].

Differences in the incidence or experience of domestic violence for pregnant women in the last 12 months in Pedungan villages and Nongan villages with

Characteristics	Village/City (N = 64 pregnant women)				*P*
	Pedungan, Denpasar (n = 31 pregnant women)		Nongan Karangasem (n = 33 pregnant women)		
	f	%	f	%	
Women education level					
Elementary	8	25.8	17	51.5	**0.008****
High school	12	38.7	14	42.4	
Diploma/university	11	35.5	2	6.1	
Partner education level					
Elementary	6	19.3	8	24.3	**0.008****
High school	15	48.4	24	72.7	
Diploma/university	10	32.3	1	3.0	
Vocational					
Yes	15	48.4	11	33.3	0.220
No	16	51.6	22	66.7	
Parity					
Primi	9	29.0	9	27.3	0.566
Multi	21	67.7	24	72.7	
Grande multi	1	3.3	0	0.0	

Source: Primary data.
* $p < 0.05$
** $p < 0.01$

Table 1.
Results of the characteristics on fertile age couples in Bali, 2015.

sociodemographic characteristics obtained that there was a significant negative correlation ($r = -0.34$) and ($p < 0.05$) between the age of the respondent or pregnant women in the village of Pedungan with a history of domestic violence in the last 12 months. This shows that if the pregnant woman gets older, the incidence of domestic violence is lower. Meanwhile, there was no significant correlation between the age of pregnant women and a history of domestic violence in the last 12 months ($p > 0.05$). The forms of violence experienced by pregnant women in the last 12 months in Pedungan Village showed that as many as 3 pregnant women admitted to experiencing physical violence in the form of: husbands throwing objects/items that are dangerous to the mother (2 people/6, 45%) and the husband threw things/objects including the mother's pet (1 person/3.23%).

In this study, the results showed that the number of women who had experienced DV in the last 12 months in Pedungan Village and in Nongan Village was not statistically different ($p > 0.05$). The number of women who had experienced DV in Nongan Village was higher than in Pedungan Village (15 people out of 33 people/45.45% vs. 10 people out of 31 people/32.26%). One in four pregnant women claimed to have been a victim of domestic violence by her husband in the last 12 months. Some respondents said there was a desire to leave their husband/partner, but this desire was rejected by parents [19]. The incidence of physical violence and sexual violence was more experienced by women in Nongan Village than in Pedungan Village (6.45% vs. 3.23%). On the other hand, incidents of sexual violence and emotional violence were mostly experienced by women in Pedungan Village [18].

The influence of traditional and religious values is very strong, especially in regions that still carry patriarchy. Women must be obedient and submit to their husbands and families [6, 7]. Almost all women who have been victims of DV in the study said that they never told others about the violence, including their family or parents. Shame, fear, and even being blamed are the main reasons women victims of violence do not share incidents of violence with others. Domestic problems are a big shame to share with others or taboo [5, 9, 10, 15, 21, 30]. This condition can worsen the situation of women. According to Kyriacou et al. (1999) suggest that women as wives are considered as the property of their husbands [25].

There is an assumption among Balinese women, that husbands have rights over women including how a woman is treated. The results obtained through self-reported questioners regarding the knowledge and attitudes of pregnant women about domestic violence, that most wives agree that a wife must always obey and follow the husband's orders. A husband can scold his wife for not obeying her wishes [19]. Women or wives in Bali still adhere to the concept of marriage, which is the embodiment of loyalty until death. The divorce process is also very difficult, because it must involve the role of traditional leaders before the court decision [2, 19, 31].

Balinese women are synonymous with individuals who obey and follow the decisions of men, especially husbands. A married Balinese woman must follow her husband, including living in a male family. In the environment where the husband lives, it is not uncommon for the wife or woman to live in an extended family, namely with the parents of the husband or in-laws, relatives of the husband or in-laws and even other family members. This condition is suspected to have triggered acts of domestic violence against women, especially wives. Balinese society in general adheres to a fatherly system (Vederrechtelijk) or in Balinese terms it is called "Purusa". The main thing that is understood from the fatherly system in Bali is the position of men as "Sentana" from the Purusa family line. The men who is the heir in the family [2, 31].

3.4 The history of physical, emotional, sexual, social and economical abuse

The problem faced by pregnant women is that the history of domestic violence that is generally experienced is not only one type, but multiple or even a pregnant woman has experienced two or more types of violence by her husband [8, 10, 17, 19]. The results obtained are that there are 2 pregnant women with a history of experiencing physical and sexual violence at the same time, there is one pregnant woman who is a victim of physical, emotional and economic violence, one person experiences sexual and social violence. As many as two pregnant women who admitted to experiencing physical and sexual violence at the same time in their lifetime, two pregnant women experienced a history of sexual and emotional violence, and the most pregnant women experienced economic violence. Thus, women at most experience more than one form of violence in their lives, especially physical, sexual and emotional violence, in addition to economic violence [19]. Women experience the most economic violence when compared to other forms of violence, such as sexual, physical, social, and emotional or psychological violence. In the picture below, an overlapping illustration of violence experienced by pregnant women in the last 12 months is shown (**Figure 1**).

The results of the study in India found that the most common type of violence reported was physical violence. The most common cause of domestic violence reported

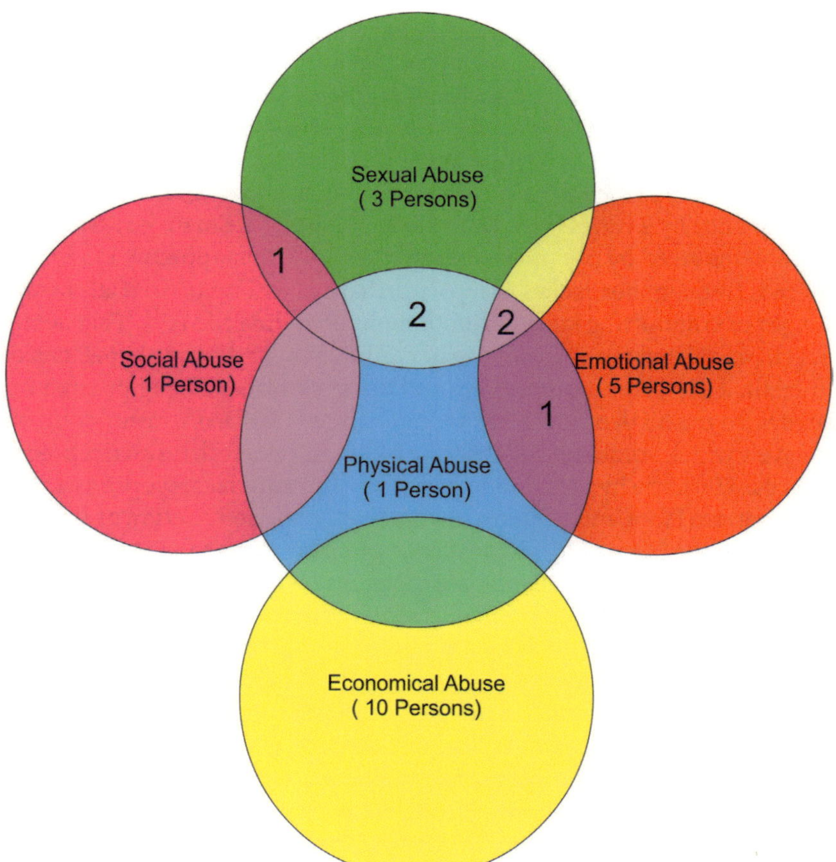

Figure 1.
Overlapping of domestic violence experience among pregnant women In Denpasar City and Karangasem Regency.

in our study was financial problems followed by influence under alcohol [32]. As many as 60% of women who reported having been threatened with violence in Uganda, but few reported acts of violence that had been experienced. The previous year, and very few reported acts of violence [9]. Thus, DV events experienced by women are in the form of more than one form of violence or multiple acts. This condition certainly has a bad impact on the health and welfare of women.

Husbands who were perpetrators of violence, when asked the reasons for beatings or engaging in sexual coercion, said that women must be educated properly by their husbands. Women must not violate the restrictions given by their husbands, as well as actions taken by their husbands as normal things to do. The explanation of this behavior is based on the WHO's ecological model framework theory. There are four levels that trigger it, namely: the individual level, personal relationships, community and societal factors. From the individual characteristics in Bali that are related to abusive behavior, they are men with low education level, low income, have a habit of drinking alcohol, live in the periphery or rural areas. Community and societal factors that trigger violence by men are patriarchal culture, family upbringing, and the existence of values that view violence is commonly committed by men. There have been no clear sanctions for perpetrators of violence. In this case, results from in-depth interviews with traditional leaders in Bali, it is found that there needs to be customary rules or "Awig-awig" for perpetrators of violence. Despite the fact, it takes a lot of hard work and a lot of money to make customary rules.

3.5 Impact of domestic violence experience to women and babies wellbeing

Pregnant women in Bali experience several forms of physical violence by their husbands, for example: beatings on the stomach, breasts and genitals which have a direct negative impact on their pregnancy [19]. In other words, the act of DV especially physical violence against pregnant women, increases the negative risk during pregnancy by 2 times [3, 4, 8, 17, 19, 25, 32–36]. The main health or psychological problems faced by pregnant women especially poor appetite, easily tired/feeling tired, frequent headaches, sleep disturbances and tired/tired all the time, had thought of committing suicide and thought of ending life [19]. That acute stress levels are related to the incidence of cardiovascular disease, hypertension, gastrointestinal disorders, chronic pain and diabetes. Stress during pregnancy is associated with the birth of low birth weight babies (LBW) as a result of increased cortisol levels which stimulate constriction of blood vessels that restrict blood flow to the uterus. Thus, the hypothalamic–pituitary-and adrenal response as a trigger or trigger of preterm labor and preterm birth, through the contraction of the smooth muscle tissue in the uterus [36]. Exposure of prenatal stress can have negative long-lasting impacts on health and disease susceptibility [4, 6–8, 19, 23, 26, 27, 34–37]. Acts of violence or abuse by an intimate partner can cause physical trauma, psychological trauma, and fear of women who are victims [38–40]. Physical trauma is experienced from mild to severe, which affects the disability and death of women. Physical disorders or trauma affect the mental health conditions of victims/women in the form of post-traumatic stress disorder, anxiety, depression, eating disorders and suicidal thoughts [3]. Sub-ordination in Bali has an impact on decision making in choosing the place of delivery, who is the delivery assistant and other preparations when facing pathological conditions and/or emergencies during pregnancy and childbirth. Decision making is mostly determined by husbands and in-laws. The wife can only be the recipient of this decision. This has an impact on delays in referral efforts and acts to save mothers and their babies, so that the morbidity and mortality rates for mothers and babies are still high.

Domestic violence is a global issue that requires extraordinary efforts from various components to overcome it. DV problem solving starts from individual, family, group and community lines. Broad-scale research in the field of gender issues, especially domestic violence, is expected to be able to open up insights and commitments from policy holders related to gender. Women who have been physically or sexually abused by their partners report higher rates of a number of important health problems [3]. According to The Legal Aid Foundation of the Indonesian Women's Association for Justice in 2020, found that strong patriarchal norms and conservative religious values that put men above women. Including the patriarchal culture in Hindu society in Bali which indirectly perpetuates acts of violence against women both in the domestic and public sphere.

3.6 Policies and roles of midwives to eliminate incidents of violence against women

The Indonesian government issued a law related to the elimination of domestic violence in 2004, which was followed by a 2009 Minister of Health decree on Guidelines for the Management of Integrated Services for Victims of Violence against Women and Children in Hospitals. The personnel or officers who have responsibility and competence in providing services to victims of violence are: 1) a forensic specialist/psychiatrist/other specialist doctor; 2) trained general practitioners; 3) midwife/nurse; 4) psychologist; 5) social workers; and 6) other health workers in the form of administrative personnel and medical records.

Midwives have a strategic role in early detection and provide assistance to pregnant women victims of violence. Midwives are health professionals who are at the forefront of maternal and child health services. Since the last decade, the issue of violence against women has been rolled out and has become a national issue. The midwife has a strategic role because pregnant women are the first to be contacted by a pregnant woman in a health care facility. Midwives with the motto as friends of women will be able to dig up more data and early detection of these incidents of violence. Screening is the right step for health workers. Screening is carried out with adequate instruments and in accordance with the local socio-culture [41].

Midwives in Bali have been given training several times regarding early detection of incidents of violence against pregnant women and referral measures, as part of integrated services in basic health care facilities. The problem is that the training activities have not been evenly distributed to all midwives on duty, so that the problem of violence against women, especially pregnant women, has not been optimally resolved. The effort of midwifery education institutions is to include the topic of gender issues and violence against women in the midwifery education curriculum, especially reproductive health. Introducing midwife students is a strategic effort as a provision in providing services in their place of duty.

Researchers in the field of reproductive health and maternal and child health have attempted to carry out various studies related to gender issues, especially the incidence of violence against women and disseminate the results of the study widely. The main obstacle in accelerating the reduction in the incidence of violence against women, especially pregnant women, is that there is no clear and sustainable policy from policy makers regarding the elimination of incidents of violence against women.

In the case in Bali, women victims of domestic violence were given explanations and were guided in efforts to save themselves and seek help when they were in a situation that threatened their safety. An important and simple trick is the most appropriate step in addition to empowering community organizations in customary villages.

4. Summary and recommendation

Balinese women are born to carry out their duties and responsibilities to become obedient, loyal and devoted women to God, ancestors, in-laws, husbands, children and their parents. That is the full responsibility of Balinese women in the family, even though sacrifice has never been properly interpreted.

Violence against women is a serious violation of human rights, because it has a negative impact on the health and welfare of women. Violence against women undermines the dignity of women as human beings. The cause of domestic violence incidents is influenced by individual, family, community and societal factors. The ecological framework of the model can explain in detail the influence of these factors on the incidence of DV. Economic abuse and emotional/psychological abuse are the most common forms of DV experienced by pregnant women in Bali. The type of abuse experienced is more of multiple abuse.

There are various reasons why health services have a critical role in helping women victims of violence. Women victims of DV will use health facilities more often, and health workers are the professionals who first make contact with victims. The most common and the most severe form of violence against women, can occur in a variety of settings. The incidence of DV is taboo to tell, in fact women are often blamed for various incidents of sexual violence they have experienced.

The role of midwives is very strategic in preventing and early detection of incidents of violence against women, especially during pregnancy, because it has a negative impact on the health and well-being of pregnant women and their fetuses. Cooperation across sectors, programs and laws and regulations that clearly regulate efforts to eliminate incidents of violence against women is urgently needed. There must be synergy between policy makers, community or traditional leaders, health care institutions and midwifery education institutions in the effort to eliminate acts of violence against women.

Acknowledgements

The author would like to thank: Head of the Health Research and Development Agency, Center for Humanities, Health Policy and Community Empowerment, Surabaya; Prof. Anom Umbara, from Udayana University as research consultant; and Prof. dr. M. Hakimi.

Conflict of interest

There was no conflict of interest in the research and preparation of this report.

Notes/thanks/other declarations

Thanks to the data analysis officers, enumerators, Mr. Akto Adi, Mr. Tri Wahyu Yuliono and respondents who played a big role in this study.

Author details

Ni Komang Yuni Rahyani*, Ni Made Dwi Mahayati,
Made Widhi Gunapria Darmapatni and Ni Wayan Armini
Polytechnique of Health of Denpasar, Midwifery Department, Ministry of Health Republic of Indonesia, Denpasar, Indonesia

*Address all correspondence to: yunirahyani@yahoo.co.id

References

[1] U. Nasaruddin and S. S. Sukri, *Bias Jender dalam Pemahaman Islam*. Yogyakarta: Pusat Studi Jender (PSJ) IAIN Walisongo dan Gama Media, 2002.

[2] I. K. Sudantra, "Wanita Bali dan Harta Benda Perkawinan: Suatu Perspektif Normatif," Jurnal Studi Gender Srikandi, vol. 2, no. 2, pp. 79-87, 2002.

[3] A. Van Parys, A. Verhamme, M. Temmerman, and H. Verstraelen, "Information sheet Intimate partner violence during pregnancy," PLoS One, vol. 9, no. 1, pp. 183-197, 2014.

[4] World Health Organization, *Global and regional estimates of violence against women: prevalence and health effects of intimate partner violence and non-partner sexual violence*. Geneva: World Health Organization, 2013.

[5] K. Alejo, "Long-term physical and mental health effects of domestic violence," *Themis: Research Journal of Justice Studies* Forensic Science, vol. 2, no. 1, p. 5, 2014.

[6] K. Åsling-Monemi, R. Pena, M. C. Ellsberg, and L. Å. Persson, "Violence against women increases the risk of infant and child mortality: a case-referent study in Nicaragua," Bulletin of the World Health Organization, vol. 81, pp. 10-16, 2003.

[7] C. García-Moreno, H. A. Jansen, M. Ellsberg, L. Heise, and C. Watts, *WHO multi-country study on women's health and domestic violence against women*. Geneva: World Health Organization, 2005.

[8] UNICEF, *Behind closed doors: The impact of domestic violence on children*. New York: UNICEF, 2006.

[9] L. Heise, M. Ellsberg, and M. Gottemoeller, "Ending violence against women," Population reports, vol. 27, no. 4, pp. 1-1, 1999.

[10] M. A. Koenig *et al.*, "Domestic violence in rural Uganda: evidence from a community-based study," Bulletin of the world health organization, vol. 81, pp. 53-60, 2003.

[11] United Nations, *The Elimination of Violence against Women*. Al-Raida, 1970.

[12] United Nations, "General Assembly Resolution 48/104 20 December 1993 Declaration on the Elimination of Violence against Women," Int J Refug Law, vol. 6, no. 4, pp. 714-718, 1994.

[13] United Nations. "Declaration on the Elimination of Violence Against Women " United Nations. http://daccess-dds-ny.un.org/doc/UNDOC/GEN/N94/095/05/PDF/N9409505.pdf?OpenElement (accessed 12 Desember, 2020).

[14] R. H. Bradley and R. F. Corwyn, "Socioeconomic status and child development," Annual review of psychology, vol. 53, no. 1, pp. 371-399, 2002.

[15] World Health Organization, "Domestic Violence Against Women and Girls," in "Innocenti Digest," World Health Organization, Geneva, 2000, vol. 1.

[16] C. García-Moreno and C. Watts, "Violence against women: an urgent public health priority," Bulletin of the World Health Organization, vol. 89, no. 2, 2011.

[17] T. Gupta and F. Samuels. "Literature review of male perpetrators of intimate partner violence in South Asia." www.odi.org/twitter (accessed 13 Desember, 2020).

[18] N. Rahyani, A. Paramita, N. Gusti, K. Sriasih, and N. Ariyani, "Events of Domestic Violence among Pregnant Women in Traditional Villages in Bali," Int J Sci Res, vol. 8, 9, pp. 1195-1198, 2019.

[19] World Health Organization. "Understanding and addressing violence against women." http://apps.who.int/iris/bitstream/10665/77434/1/WHO_RHR_12.37_ eng. pdf (accessed 4 Desember, 2020).

[20] H. Douglas and K. Chapple, *National domestic and family violence bench book*. Brisbane, Australia: Australasian Institute of Judicial Administration, 2017.

[21] A. L. Ganley, "Understanding domestic violence," in *Improving the health care response to domestic violence: A resource manual for health care providers*, L. Ganley, J. Fazio, A. Hyman, L. James, and A. Ruiz-Contreras Eds. San Francisco, CA: The Family Violence Prevention Fund, 1995, pp. 15-42.

[22] EuroHealthNet. "Making the link: Gender Equality and Health." https://eurohealthnet.eu/sites/eurohealthnet.eu/files/publications/PP_Gender_Digital%20 Version.pdf (accessed 3 Desember, 2020).

[23] J. Walsh, J. Spangaro, and K. Soldatic, "Global understandings of domestic violence," Nursing and Health Sciences, pp. 1-4, 2015.

[24] E. Coutinho, F. Almeida, J. Duarte, C. Chaves, P. Nelas, and O. Amaral, "Factors related to domestic violence in pregnant women," Procedia-Social and Behavioral Sciences, vol. 171, pp. 1280-1287, 2015.

[25] D. N. Kyriacou *et al.*, "Risk factors for injury to women from domestic violence," New England journal of medicine, vol. 341, no. 25, pp. 1892-1898, 1999.

[26] World Health Organization. "Intimate partner violence during pregnancy." https://apps.who.int/iris/bitstream/handle/10665/70764/WHO_RHR_11.35_eng.pdf;jsessionid=6EDFDE8E9E464356E7B8FAD11D3F967D?sequence=1 (accessed 12 Desember, 2020).

[27] World Health Organization, "Health care for women subjected to intimate partner violence or sexual violence: A clinical handbook," World Health Organization, Geneva, 2014.

[28] World Health Organization, "Global plan of action: health systems address violence against women and girls," World Health Organization, Geneva, 2016.

[29] UNFPA. "New survey shows violence against women widespread in Indonesia." https://www.unfpa.org/news/new-survey-shows-violence-against-women-wides pread-indonesia (accessed 13 Desember, 2020).

[30] M. Alam and M. Islam, "Factors Affecting Domestic Violence against Women in Bangladesh," European Journal of Public Health, vol. 25, no. 3, 2015.

[31] K. Hemamalini and U. Suhardi, "Dinamika Perkawinan Adat Bali: Status dan Kedudukan Anak Sentana Rajeg Menurut Hukum Adat dan Hukum Hindu," *Dharmasmrti*, XIII, vol. 26, pp. 36-47, 2015.

[32] A. K. Jawarkar, H. Shemar, V. R. Wasnik, and M. S. Chavan, "Domestic violence against women: a crossectional study in rural area of Amravati district of Maharashtra, India," International Journal of Research in Medical Sciences, vol. 4, no. 7, pp. 2713-2718, 2016.

[33] T. Abramsky *et al.*, "What factors are associated with recent intimate partner violence? Findings from the WHO multi-country study on women's health and domestic violence," BMC public health, vol. 11, no. 1, p. 109, 2011.

[34] B. A. Bailey, "Partner violence during pregnancy: prevalence, effects, screening, and management," International journal of women's health, vol. 2, p. 183, 2010.

[35] J. Devaney, "Research Review: The Impact of Domestic Violence on Children," *Irish probation journal,* vol. 12, 2015.

[36] S. Entringer, C. Buss, and P. D. Wadhwa, "Prenatal stress, development, health and disease risk: A psychobiological perspective—2015 Curt Richter Award Paper," Psychoneuroendocrinology, vol. 62, pp. 366-375, 2015.

[37] K. D. Pun *et al.*, "Domestic violence and perinatal outcomes–a prospective cohort study from Nepal," BMC public health, vol. 19, no. 1, p. 671, 2019.

[38] F. Abdollahi, F. R. Abhari, M. A. Delavar, and J. Y. Charati, "Physical violence against pregnant women by an intimate partner, and adverse pregnancy outcomes in Mazandaran Province, Iran," Journal of family & community medicine, vol. 22, no. 1, pp. 13-18, 2015.

[39] Z. Tavoli, A. Tavoli, R. Amirpour, R. Hosseini, and A. Montazeri, "Quality of life in women who were exposed to domestic violence during pregnancy," BMC pregnancy and childbirth, vol. 16, no. 1, pp. 1-7, 2016.

[40] A. Tiwari *et al.*, "The impact of psychological abuse by an intimate partner on the mental health of pregnant women," BJOG: An International Journal of Obstetrics & Gynaecology, vol. 115, no. 3, pp. 377-384, 2008.

[41] H. D. Nelson, C. Bougatsos, and I. Blazina, "Screening women for intimate partner violence: a systematic review to update the US Preventive Services Task Force recommendation," Annals of internal medicine, vol. 156, no. 11, pp. 796-808, 2012.

Chapter 12

Poverty, Reproductive Health and Public Health Policies in Chile

Estela Arcos Griffiths

Abstract

In Chile the social inequality is the result of the accumulation and concentration of income, wealth and property coming from the prevailing neoliberal model in the chilean economy. Under this model, persistent gaps in basic living standards, precarious assets, disparities in health, and inequalities in well-being, employment, treatment and safety of people have been configured. Using the case study methodology, evidence of the phenomenon is presented, making an analysis of the expression of poverty and other social determinants in the results of the reproductive health of socially vulnerable women. Scientific literature on the situation of exclusion and invisibility of subgroups of women who have experienced domestic violence, unplanned pregnancy, early motherhood, migration and ethnic status is analyzed. In turn, the results of effective transfers of health and social benefits to women in social adversity are mentioned in the management of health policy and the social protection system. Finally, a reflection is presented on the need for innovation in the processes of human capital formation in health and social science, and as a response, strategies are proposed to address it to from the complexity of the phenomenon of vulnerability and inequality in reproductive health analyzed.

Keywords: poverty, reproductive health, public health, vulnerability, reproductive rights

1. Introduction

Equity is not synonymous with equality, because equality means to give value to the inequalities, from the idea of justice, therefore, this premise demands a social epidemiological approach to value inequities and inequalities as health problems determinants [1]. Health equity implies, ideally, that everyone should have the opportunity to attain their full health potential and no one should be excluded to reach such potential [1]. This equity is then defined as equality of access to the health care comparing the same needs; equality in the use of resources for the same needs; equality of quality of care and equality of health results [2, 3]. Disparities and inequalities in health are an objective expression of the socioeconomic disadvantage accumulated by the individuals throughout their lifetime, which should be prevented with timely intervention strategies, where the intensity and duration of which would vary according to the degree of vulnerability [4]. The scientific literature has given a fund of evidence about the influence that the social determinants have on the individual and familiar health, as the substratum of diverse illnesses that manifest regardless the universal access that people may have to health systems [5, 6]. The social inequality is the result of the accumulation and concentration of incomes, wealth and property coming from the prevailing neoliberal model in the Chilean economy [7–10]. Under this model have raised public, economic, political and social policies [9], which have set a new generation of inequalities expressed in persistent gaps in the basic living standards, the precariousness of assets, negatively affected emotional ties and solidarity, health disparities and inequalities regarding well-being, jobs, treatment and security of people in their communities [8, 11–15].

Currently, Chile is recognized as the Latin American country with the highest human development index (HDI), according data of 2020 (0.851), the lowest poverty rate and one of the highest levels of per capita income in the region [11, 15]. The country is in the world's 62nd place in the Gender Development Index (GDI) and 39nd place in Gender Index scores about 2019 across 129 countries, at the same time, has one of the highest inequality rates in Latin America, being the country with the most inequality of the Organization for Economic Cooperation and Development [16, 17]. When we consider the inequality as a result of the inequality of incomes, education and health, the country fall 11 places in the world's ranking, falling to the 54th place (Chile's HDI falls from 0.851 to 0.709) [15]. Considering this context, the chilean society shows and keeps deep inequalities, inequities and differences that generate a sense of growing frustration, mistrust and social unrest in the population [14, 18–19].

2. Methodology

To address the situation of poverty, inequality, reproductive health, a case study is carried out to understand the how and why of the causes and consequences of the phenomena that occurred in Chile, unit of analysis, regarding the subject under study. The case study corresponds to an empirical investigation based on a set of heterogeneous evidences in its origin and that converge in the explanation of a set of contemporary phenomena that arise in real life regarding poverty, inequality, reproductive health and public policies. Objective methods of searching for evidence are used through repositories of university databases and Chilean and international public organizations. The foregoing is complemented with information from studies carried out by the author with a team of researchers who approached the research on the subject in question in particular groups and territories and that account for the knowledge generated in the field work.

Finally, three strategies are presented for the development of competencies and skills in transdisciplinary and integrated management practices in primary health care for midwifery students and academics and student from other health and social science careers-professions.

3. Poverty, inequality and disparity in reproductive health: evidences about the Chilean case

The concept of health inequalities has been defined as "the differences that in health are not only unnecessary and avoidable, but also are considered unfair" [20–23] and, inequity is considered as any reducible difference or inequality, related to heterogeneous life conditions tied up with incomes differences, even when the poorest have equality of access to health services [21, 24, 25]. The perspective of social, cultural and political determinants of health has allowed to understand the mechanism underlying as substratum in the "causes of the causes" and in the routes or production processes of the inequities [22, 26]. That is how it is detected the interaction between health and the social circumstances within the area where people live, where poverty has been described as the most potentially toxic risk factor for the population health, effect which shows from early ages, reproduce during adult life and transfer to following generations [10, 23, 24, 27]. Scientific evidences have demonstrated that there is a relation between the income gap between rich and poor and the mortality rate and physical and mental health problems [10, 28], which affects the possibilities and opportunities for people development. There is an unequal distribution of the mortality rate in Chile, because the child mortality in children born to mothers with no education have significantly lower survival rates than those born to mothers with secondary or higher education [29]. Is one of the reasons that justifies that medicine alone cannot solve people's health problems, since 56% of the variations of health conditions are explained by social and ecological factors [23, 30].

The condition of women is a political, economic, and social issue and the inequalities registered must be explained by social, economic, and cultural phenomenon [31]. The inequality consists of a systematic exclusion from power, resources, and opportunities [17, 31]. The attempt to identify the factors that explain women social and economic vulnerability should start examining first the impact of developing models, and some of their components, on the gender social inequalities [31].

In the 1960s, the standard of living of the richest and the poorest people was compared and it turned out that the poor lived thirty times worse than the rich. At the end of the 1990s, the poor already lived eighty-two times worse than the rich. The differences between the rich and the poor are constantly increasing. They appear already on a family level, but they are also reflected on the fate of children and, especially, women. The efforts to visualize the inequalities between men and women are more recent [17]. The study of differentiated impacts that economic policies on men and women have had, and currently have, has demonstrated that regardless of women's social group, they have created a continue discrimination of women compared to their male colleagues [17]. The income distribution is based on an imposed cultural contract, which highly values motherhood and naturalizes the unpaid domestic work of women.

Global incomes separated by sex show that, although the gap is growing [19], the earning capacity remains minor for women, while their contribution to the reproduction continues in the dark statistics [32]. There is a welfare and mercantilist concept of the economic models that create a strong "feminization of poverty" and exclusion of the incorrectly called "ethnic minorities". Women represent an increasing percentage of those people considered to be poor. In a world that is heading towards the globalization, women's poverty creates enclaves of people in need in the midst of wealth and originates growing pressure on the developed world, whether generating expensive humanitarian crisis or trigger--for the first time in history--a surge of women migrating without their husbands and children to look for a job in richest countries, which has a significant impact in the family and society. The available evidence suggests that the proportion of poor is higher among the family groups with a female head of the household, especially when the woman has small children. In Latin America, single female-headed families are largest in the category of low incomes (homeless) [33].

Regarding reproductive health, women's greater social vulnerability and economic precariousness during pregnancy is associated to higher stress levels and anxiety and, as a consequence, higher incidence of prematurity, low birth weight, early weaning, poor child care quality, higher rates of disadvantage, child developmental delay, poor child care quality, attention deficit and hyperactivity, language problems, poor social competences and lifelong behavior problems, which is the first link in the transmission and reproduction of inequalities of health, welfare and human capital [34–36]. In addition, it has been pointed out that coronary heart disease, type 2 diabetes, vascular accidents, hypertension, and higher rates of adult mortality are related to the history of fetal malnutrition and low birth weight [35]. Moreover, the reproductive, neonatal, mental, and family health deteriorate when women have precarious employments and pregnancies without social security, informal and insecure houses, low schooling, psychosocial risk, absence of partner at home and high dependency rate [35].

In Chile, through surveys performed in vulnerable women's groups, it was possible to obtain an in-depth knowledge of the experience of motherhood in extreme vulnerability conditions [37]. The women's stories showed a motherhood perceived as a negative event, unexpected, assumed with resignation and anguish which, for some authors, generate internal disorganization, break of bonds and depression [37]. Feelings such as discomfort, despair and loneliness emerged, both for being an unforeseen pregnancy and for being unexpected and that is consistent with the precariousness of the social support to teach women on how to take care in a context of social vulnerability [37, 38]. Women describe a life condition where the social construction of hopelessness, invisibility and social exclusion have been naturalized, a condition which affects the practice of motherhood, childcare and sexual and reproductive rights [37, 39]. The situation of invisibility is not an isolated fact, because it occurs in a condition of poverty with a gender perspective. Women perceive a distance between them and health personnel, which they feel as lack of understanding of their condition of vulnerability and poverty, due to the asymmetrical power relations and stigmatization of guilty for their pregnancy [39]. The more difficult it is for a woman to carry out motherhood and children care, the further she is from a project that justify the exercise of her reproductive rights [40, 41].

In the context of reproductive health and poverty, some relevant facts for women are domestic violence (DV), unplanned pregnancy, immigrant status, Mapuche ethnicity and teenage motherhood.

3.1 Violence against women

Is a global public health problem [42] and its prevalence is higher in developing countries [43]. Pregnancy is an especially vulnerable period in terms of violence, affecting women's reproductive capacity [44], since pregnant women have an increased risk than no pregnant women [45]. Prevalence studies about DV have reported figures varying from 0,9% to 41,6,0%, being more severe or moderate post birth [42, 46]. One out of every five pregnant teenage women and one out of every six pregnant adult women have reported violent experiences during pregnancy. Violence during pregnancy becomes four times probable if the pregnancy was unexpected or unplanned [47].

The impact of domestic violence on the results of reproductive and neonatal health may be explained by the existence of indirect mechanisms that induce risks like psychological and social stress, which would be like underlying factors of adverse obstetric and neonatal results. It has been reported that biomedical risks, for women with experience of domestic violence, are related to pregnancy hypertensive states (PHS), intra-hepatic cholestasis of pregnancy (ICP), and in case of current violence with urinary tract infection, intrauterine growth restriction, preterm delivery and ICP [48]. Other associated risks are poor weight gain, vaginal, cervical or kidney infections, abdominal trauma, bleeding, exacerbation of chronic diseases, complications during labor, delay in the prenatal care, depression, suicide attempt and, even death [42, 43, 46]. At the same time, violence determines disturbances in the interaction between mother and son, which increases the possibility of negligence, abuse and neglect during the first year of life. The Biomedical risks for neonatal health related to domestic violence are low rate of gestational age, and higher variability of anthropometric indicators such as weight and length at birth. It was observed 2.8 higher risk of small for gestational age newborns in relation to those of women without recognizing experiences of violence [48].

3.2 Unplanned pregnancy

Regarding unplanned pregnancy, it is observed that in high-income countries half of the pregnancies are unplanned, which increases sanitary costs for women care, originates personal and family crisis for women and commits timely health care [49, 50]. In the period 2015–2019, there were 121.0 million of unwanted pregnancies per year, which represent a rate of 64 unwanted pregnancies for every 1000 women between 15 to 49 years old. Out of the total, a 61.0% of the unwanted pregnancies resulted in abortion, that is to say, a global rate of 39 abortions per 1000 women. The rates of unwanted pregnancies are higher in countries where abortion is illegal [51]. It is pointed out that 63 million of these unwanted pregnancies are, at least, consequence that 22 million women around the world have an unsatisfied need of family planning [49, 52]. In the United States 50% of pregnancies are unplanned, a 50% result in abortion and increases women's depression and 47.0% of the live births come from an unplanned pregnancy [50, 53].

In Chile, in the five-year period of 2010, the unplanned pregnancy represented a 51,0% out the total of the pregnant entered to the public health system, prenatal care, higher in the extreme age groups, reaching an 85.6% in pregnant under 15 years old and a 66% in older than 45 years old [54]. In the United States, there are disparities in the rates of unwanted pregnancies between poor and non-poor women, being the rate 5 times higher in the first group [25]. In addition, Also, pregnancy disparities have been observed regarding unplanned pregnancies in the poor women subgroups of 18 to 24 years old or who cohabit with a partner, since they have twice or three times the national rate [55, 56]. It is possible that the unplanned pregnancy is related to social naturalization of motherhood, in addition to the access difficulties and the lack of information about the fertility regulation means [56, 57].

Timely access to health centers in order to search early for pregnancies is very important for women who did not plan a pregnancy, since they find out 2 weeks later than women with wanted pregnancies. Fetal organs are formed at the 8th week, so a 2-week delay further than the normal 6 weeks' recognition period could prevent a form taking fast responses regarding reproductive health, especially in women with unwanted pregnancies. The possible effect of unhealthy behaviors, such as smoking and drinking, could be continuously unnoticed during the embryonic period, when most of the malformations occur [57]. It has been reported that women from minority ethnic groups have noticed very late, compared to white non-Hispanic women, since they have less information about family planning and less access to health care [57, 58]. The evidence show that unplanned pregnancy is related to disparities in women health and perinatal health in relation to the late prenatal care: low birth weight, child abuse and negligence, child behavior problems, exposure risk to illicit drugs or tobacco, not preventing alterations due to not taking folic acid timely, high prevalence of depression, depression during pregnancy and postpartum [52, 59, 60].

3.3 Inmigrant pregnant women

Illegal immigrant pregnant women constitute a socially vulnerable group, since they have legal limitations to access to prenatal and obstetric care to protect their health and their children's health [52, 61]. Scientific evidence demonstrate that immigrant women's reproductive health is exposed to a high rate of unplanned pregnancies, pregnancy rejection and late prenatal care. It is possible that the access difficulties and the lack of information about the fertility regulation means predispose women to unplanned pregnancy in this group [56, 57]. The possible effect of unhealthy behaviors, such as smoking and drinking, could be unnoticed during the embryonic period, when most of the malformations occur [58]. Inadequate prenatal health care to migrant women has as consequence 4 times more risk to give birth children with low birth weight and seven times more risk of prematurity [61].

3.4 Maternity in adolescent women

Regarding early motherhood, it has been informed that when reproductive timing has been examined in teenager women who start their sexual life early, the results show that teenagers with subsequent children with short/long gestational intervals belong to social groups differentiated by structural and cultural determinations. In poor women, early motherhood is considered as a non- normative crisis that determines reproductive inequity and, in some cases, excess of unwanted fertility [62, 63]. Within this framework, the concern about what happens with teenage pregnancy is not only based on studies on pregnancy rate trends and biomedical morbidity, but also on the consequences of sexual and reproductive behavior pattern and its path on education, work, and family life after delivery [63, 64]. In developing countries, longitudinal follow-up studies of teenage mothers have observed that the mother-son binomial is a strong candidate to lead-up to poverty from one generation to the next one, especially when the father is absent, because in addition to producing economic deprivation it has a negative effect on the child's socialization process [63, 65]. The disadvantage situation of the adolescent mother tends to be repeat harder on her daughter, who shows school problems and become pregnant earlier than her mother the reproductive and sexual behavior perpetuated [66].

3.5 Motherhood in ethnic groups

Finally, some reflections on poverty and reproductive health of women from Mapuche ethnicity. In Chile, poverty and marginalization are eminently rural and affect, mostly, to the regions with a highest proportion of rural and indigenous population [67]. In a study carried out in a rural area of southern Chile, a social reality of accumulated disadvantages and a situation of vulnerability was observed in Mapuche's women whose determinants of the inequity and discrimination were gender (woman), ethnicity (indigenous), class (poverty) and territory (rural) [68]. Many of the health risks of indigenous women were directly related to their reproductive health, since they had a high fertility rate, early motherhood, short birth interval and poor access to family planning services [68]. Another study analyzed the relative risk (RR) concepts of perinatal mortality and the findings revealed a direct relation between maternal poverty of Mapuche's women and perinatal mortality [69].

4. Public health policy management

There is concrete evidence that gender stereotypes are maintained and naturalized in health policies and programs [70]. Women's health programs have paid more attention to aspects related to reproductive health rather than to reproductive rights [71]. Everyday life elements present in people's life style has been rescued and put in a leading role by promotion and prevention programs, however, they are partially included in the institutional practice.

Regarding the health care providers and the female users of the public health network, the trend is to regulate the habits, modify beliefs and cancel the explanations reports by women. That is, it is excluded people's social dimension and cultural meanings [71]. Consultant women tend to inform their cases relating their symptom's to diverse aspects of their daily lives, as well as with their own opinions and beliefs about what is happening to them. For their part, health professionals emphasize objectivity and the separation between the subject who knows and the objects that are known, they tend to direct the conversation in strictly clinical terms, without allowing women to express themselves as they wish. Professionals decide what issues are appropriate and what not to manage the context of the interview. This hierarchical relationship is exacerbated in case of lower-class women and represents the fundamental asymmetry that explains many of the disagreements between providers and female users. This form of social interaction categorizes the human reproduction as a biological event, which establishes the basis to exclude the contextualization [72].

It is in these poverty contexts, where the challenge is generated for midwifery professionals to open a space to make effective the sexual and reproductive rights and, as a consequence, to modify the inequalities relationships in the reproduction and sexual day-to-day labour. This space gives an opportunity for midwives and social science professionals to give an integrated contribution to acknowledge the existing bonds between the women's health condition and the socially structured environments where they live. The changes required in the models and processes of "how to do, with what and whom with" are due to the scenarios of deep and complex social transformations generated by the growing social inequality [73, 74]. Due to the above mentioned, it is imperative to give better and greater attention to the poorest, most vulnerable, and unprotected groups, not only to strengthen prevention and promote skills that allow them their sexual and reproductive rights, but also to facilitate resilience, personal and family psycho-social development and respect for their social rights [37]. On the other hand, from the lessons learned in the Primary Health Care, the evaluation of the effectiveness of the transfer benefits of the social programs is key in the development of capabilities in the integrated management of the Primary Health Care level and from the intersector, because they are in a privilege position to take the challenge and commitment to guarantee the access to benefits to vulnerable people [75].

The general and local social, economic and political situation deserves to make balances and permanent checking on the sexual and reproductive health management to primary health level as a way to keep a dialog among the different institutions in charge to execute preventive convergent policies. In this balance, social and human capital women's in vulnerable societies require leaders that create bonds, trust, and social networks to construct synergy processes where the appreciation and mutual respect coexist [76]. Due this, it is urgent a permanent strengthening of female and male midwives as managers and executors of humanized reproductive health policy and social protection, increase the etno-cultural knowledge, apply gender perspective in health practice, streghthen management in integrated network and participate in the local analysis of integrated information systems [76].

5. How to reduce the consequences of social inequality on the results of reproductive health in socially vulnerable women's?

It has already been noted that income inequalities contribute to health inequality, regardless of universal access to health systems. In addition, it has been noted that Chile has one of the greater concentrations of wealth and one of the higher levels of inequality the world [77]. Social, economic, cultural and politic determinants had allowed to understand the mechanism underlying the production processes of these health inequalities. Therefore, estimating that reducing the adverse consequences of reproductive health could be remedied through the distribution of wealth is a true possibility, but for a very long term and practically utopian in the developing countries.

The mitigation of the poor results in reproductive health in poor communities, must focus on the changes required by the segmented and fragmented health practice, both in health programs as well as in social programs. The best practices for an integrated management are reached through the articulation of activities and fluid relations between disciplines, professions, departments, institutions, and organizations [78]. Thus, it is overcome the ambivalence of the responsibilities and the institutional segmentation in the execution of the reproductive health policy, among other [79].

Reality shows that the construction of disciplinary knowledge has been performed through activities governed by models and/or paradigms that organize the thinking and mutilated vision of reality. In Chile, midwives working in primary health care recognize poor skills to address complex social problems that affect women's healthy [80, 81]. The health practice has been developed excessively segmented and without communication, which is a culture of fragmented work that just benefits to those who apply specific perspectives and do not solve collective issues of greater social complexity. The fragmentation is the heart of ineffectiveness because it determines a poor link between health systems and social systems [79]. To achieve an approximation to what people, require an accurate diagnosis is needed, which must necessarily represent the psychosocial reality of the groups with which we will work and, have as much knowledge as possible of the forms of solution from people's own perspectives, of what they recognize as problems and what they want as a solution.

For this reason, the opportunity to take on the task is an ethical and social responsibility imperative. Today it is required to assume a transdisciplinary approach as a form of cooperation among the different disciplines, since health problems are extraordinarily complex, and their study can just be performed through the convergence and combination of different perspectives [82]. The interaction between the disciplines results on an intercommunication and mutual enrichment with a transformation of research methodologies, fundamental concepts and terminologies modification. There is a balance of power in the established relations, where the teamwork negotiation facilitates all sorts of clarifications and debates about methodological, conceptual, and ideological issues [83]. Transdisciplinary promotes the development of skills related to complex thinking, divergent thinking, adaptability, sensitivity to other people, risk acceptance, acceptance of diversity and new roles in integrated management networks.

In this scenario, the challenge for the professional empowerment for midwifery is related to changes in the pre- and postgraduate training of midwives. It begins in a transformative process with innovations and relevance in the design of educational practices linked to behaviors and social changes, for the generation of competencies and capacities of human capital with a gender and transdisciplinary perspective [84, 85]. The gender perspective allows work teams to eliminate stereotypes as a substrate of gender inequality, stigma and prejudice and the transdisciplinary perspective facilitates the understanding of the entire network of interactions and contradictions that occur between the different phenomena, where the complexity and uncertainty of the results of an action prevail [84, 85]. The observation and analysis of the social reality of health through transdiscipline breaks with the barriers of static and intolerant professional profiles, to rethink knowledge from a cognitive continuum in which one dialogs and constructs collectively, to overcome disparities and inequality in reproductive health among socially vulnerable women [86].

In short, both for public policy managers and in the health and social sciences academia, the biomedical and medicalized model must be complemented by the psychosocial model by the complexity of interactions between biological,

DOI: http://dx.doi.org/10.5772/intechopen.96100

psychological, and socio-cultural components that health problems have. The optimization of qualitative results at the primary level of health care requires examining and reflecting on how problems are constituted, contextualizing the individual and collective social reality, defining its territoriality, and then building, together with the care subjects, a collective strategy that enhances the assets and strategies of action of women, families, households, and community group. For the systemic resolution of complex problems, the formation of competencies and skills of a relevant and effective health practice using a sequenced combination in three strategic axes is essential: a) selection of critical cases that induce critical, reflective, and creative thinking with integrative work methodologies. Creativity is the ability to think, produce and act innovatively in the various fields of social action; b) Case study with advice and monitoring of inclusive and simultaneous work with students of careers in Health, Law, Informatics, Sociology and Anthropology, among others, to incorporate methodological procedures that allow them to recognize the assets and liabilities of women-families-households and communities and to define territorial areas with vulnerability and social exclusion and, c) Training academics in problem-based learning methodologies, problem solving, evidence-based medicine and communication and expression implemented in an educational practice focused on learning. This strategy generates synergy in the social and cultural construction of knowledge, improves understanding from the perspective of the other and achieves learning situated in the social reality where the experiences of life and health of women are realized. Also, the ability to tolerate diversity, appreciate the points of view of others (intellectual empathy), collaborate in a productive way in a group, and communicate their thinking will be strengthened in future professionals. In this way, the resolution capacity of transdisciplinary teams is improved, which is the way to overcome the segmentation and fragmentation of public management in reproductive health, and, as a result, to ensure the delivery of timely and relevant support to the vulnerable population.

6. Management proposals for the development of competencies and skills in integrated health practice

6.1 Building alliances from transdisciplinarity for the integrated care of reproductive health

A management model is designed for the process of transferring benefits from programs linked to the Social Protection Network in a public family health center located in a territorial area with highly socially vulnerable neighborhoods. The design of the management model takes as reference the following assumptions i) service providers and students in practice, from health and social sciences careers, have a partial view of the social reality and lack of knowledge of the social determinants affecting the health and reproductive health of women with a history of early motherhood, unplanned pregnancy, domestic violence, immigrant women, women of the Mapuche ethnic group; ii) complexity and diversity of social dynamics; iii) low level of knowledge of public social protection policy; iv) fragmentation of work at the primary level of health care and, with the intersector; v) fragmentation of institutional databases; vi) basic capabilities for the processing and analysis of databases of the Red Protege in health centers and local government departments; and vii) value dilemmas, the social commitment and accumulated experience of the work teams. For this reason, the management model is created with the work teams involved, because the endogenous development of the change processes, accompanied by experts, facilitates the adoption of innovations, and minimizes resistance to change. The design and implementation will be carried out in a process that is structured in four axes:

i. To "literate" teams on the socio-cultural context and social determinants, based on evidence from the target population.

ii. Training in the content and foundations of public policy on social protection, ethics, and social commitment.

iii. Development of integrated working practices, use of participatory methodologies, formulation of learning strategies, design of manuals, guides and protocols according to the contents of the associated programmes of the Social Protection Network.

iv. Design of the monitoring and systematization process of benefit transfer records.

Participation in the intervention will be voluntary and the decision will be made by the woman once she knows the objectives, its procedures, is able to assess its costs and benefits, her questions are answered and explain the content of the Informed Consent Act for signature.

The design, implementation and application are represented in a process flow diagram (**Figure 1**).

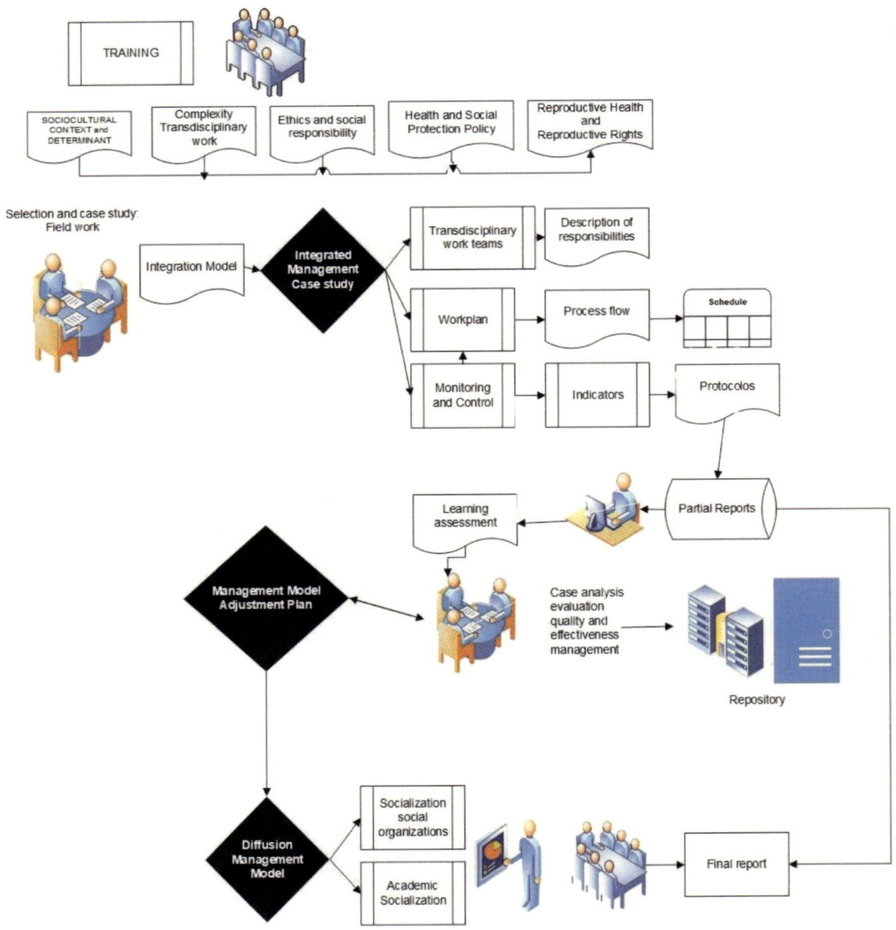

Figure 1.
Management of integrated processes in reproductive health in primary health care.

6.2 Model for promoting of sexual and reproductive rights in rural women

Women living in rural areas socialize their lives in an environment where there is no stimulus. This kind of socialization has perpetuated a condition of procrastination, subordination, inequality, and exclusion that make the practice of the exercise of sexual and reproductive rights unfeasible, as set out in the Cairo Plan of Action and the Beijing World Women's Conference. On the other hand, the institutional social resources responsible for the promotion of these rights, for various reasons, have not been effective in managing to position women as subjects of right in the definition of their sexual and reproductive life. The proposed Active Communication Strategy Model for Rural Women (MECAR) is a complementary instruction/information alternative that seeks to promote the empowerment of rural women around the exercise of sexual and reproductive rights.

The challenge of opening a space for the effective exercise of sexual and reproductive rights and, as a consequence, to modify relations of inequality in the work of reproduction and sexuality opens up a possibility, for health and social sciences professionals and students, to contribute to the recognition of the links between women's health status and the socially structured environments in which women live.

MECAR model objectives:

- To recognize socio-cultural traits; level of knowledge, beliefs, and practices of sexual and reproductive rights; characterize power relations in the couple and family; define the type of functioning and conflicts of the family, parenting models and social support networks for rural women.

- To know the types and forms of use of the media of the population subject to the intervention.

- To design a communication model for the promotion and exercise of sexual and reproductive rights based on the manifest and latent needs of women in a selected rural community.

- To know the institutional context of norms, perceptions, and information level of health service providers regarding human rights, sexual rights, reproductive rights, sexual and reproductive health concepts and women's health program content before and after the intervention.

- To know the types and forms of use of women's health services related to sexual and reproductive health, in official and alternative health centers, before and after the intervention.

- To know and compare the conditions of access, availability, and degree of use of services by rural women before and after the intervention

- Dimension the impact of the intervention on the awareness and practice of human rights, sexual rights, and reproductive rights; family functioning; power relations in the family.

Expected result of MECAR: To obtain an approach to the degree of change and contribution that MECAR produces to the process of strengthening women's self-management and self-determination to begin the path that will allow them to assume their condition as subjects of rights responsible for their life project.

Methodology: the intervention, MECAR, uses the sequenced combination of a communication strategy and interactive sessions as complementary alternatives to education on sexual and reproductive rights. The idea is to apply the model generated from the customs and traditions of the rural women's population, respecting the idiosyncrasies of their socio-cultural context, also incorporating official and traditional health resources.

MECAR has two essential components: instruction/information actions aimed at promoting reproductive rights and sexual rights for rural women, and instruction/information actions for the health team and formal and informal health leaders. A transdisciplinary team will implement instruction/information activities through a communication strategy and group workshops and analysis meetings with women, health care providers and other local leaders (active strategy).

The model operates through the following thematic axes: Gender Concept and Relations; Communication and Identity; Safe Shared Sexuality and Motherhood; Constitutional, Legal and Human Rights; Reproductive Rights and Reproductive Health; Family Planning; Prevalent and Emerging Diseases of Women; Sexually Transmitted Diseases; Adolescence and Sexuality; Women's Program Health Services; Prevention and Consequences of Physical Abuse; Family and Parenting, Role of Mother and Father, Community Participation and Leadership, and Creation; Legal protection against actions of violation of rights.

The contents will be developed in 16 radio modules and reinforced with group workshops, using active, participatory, experiential, and reflective methodology, which has as its central axis the commitment of the person, their experiences and learning of life. This methodology provides the only opportunity for participants to discover their own knowledge and the ability to learn new and diverse content related to the situation they face. The activities will be implemented with teaching-learning modules that allow women to replicate them in their family and community context. Each module will have predefined objectives, themes and methodology in which practical and theoretical activities will be combined. An important component of each module is the evaluation process because it allows for feedback to the program. The symbology and codes used in the module design are adapted to the population receiving the intervention.

In parallel, training activities are carried out for professionals and students in gender relations, reproductive health and sexuality; human rights, sexual and reproductive rights; quality of provider-user interaction for health service providers, doctors, midwives, dentists, nurses, paramedical assistants, administrative and service personnel, with monitoring and evaluation of baseline behaviors before and after the application of the training, in order to contrast the responses they are able to give to behavior change in the population of participating women.

In the field, a simultaneous examination of family and community factors and resources that may facilitate or interfere with women's health-related behaviors is conducted. This will prepare the health team and students for the potential increase in demand for health services. In harmony with this model, the people who carry out the activities will establish a dialogical communication with the women to create a link in the community.

6.3 High complexity case study: problem-based learning construction

It offers a space for reflection and practice of a contextualized, integrated, and flexible learning model based on problematic situations where the student defines strategies for the autonomous and collective construction of knowledge.

In this proposal, the sequential combination of three axes is used:

a. Analysis of critical cases that induce critical thinking, reflective-conscious learning and debate using integrative work methodologies

b. Fieldwork, consultancy and monitoring for the development of work competencies in the being, knowledge, know-how, and know-how to be in undergraduate students, community agents and officials of the intra and intersectoral.

c. Training in constructivist methodologies of collective learning with a gender perspective, application of qualitative methodologies and social vulnerability approach, problem solving, evidence-based health care, communication-expression, and leadership.

For the first axis: An educational strategy is proposed that combines educational methodological resources related to cognitive, operational, and social relationship and interaction. Activities are proposed to strengthen skills in the use of conventional system records, interviews with program supervisors, professionals, and officials. Activities are planned with groups of women, affected by similar health problems, to learn the opinions and meanings they give to their problems and ways of solving them. Participant observation, field work, individual interviews with women. Joint presentation of the analysis of critical situations in a round table with the participation of experts Training and monitoring activities for the use of resource networks such as: data banks and networks, documentary networks, project banks, scientific cooperation networks, governmental and non-governmental community resources. The integrated participation of students from schools of the Faculty of Medicine, Law, Informatics and Anthropology, community agents, specialists and officials are considered.

For the second axis, transdisciplinary systems of field work, consultancy and monitoring are implemented, both individually and collectively, according to the profile of the problems to be addressed. A cadastre of access systems is configured, as well as a map of methodological, information and social resources that will be located on a university server site.

The third axis consists of a training program expressed in seven workshops: Incorporation of the gender perspective at work, Social Vulnerability Approach, Application of qualitative methodologies for the contextualization of the social reality, Problem-based learning, Evidence-based health care, Communication-Expression, and Leadership. For the execution of these workshops there are specialists convened by invitation. Also considered is the idea of convening teams from other centers, from the intersector, to enhance the multiplier effect of the workshops. For the execution of the workshops, we count on the facilities of the primary health centers of the public network.

7. Conclusion

Finally, to mitigate the consequences of the growing social inequalities in reproductive health and reproductive rights, an integrated management of professionals from all social sectors is urgently needed, with networking and active community participation. It is necessary to broaden the view of reproductive health actions, understood as a network of meanings and interactions, in which women's behaviors are configured in a diversity of sociocultural, psychoaffective and political contexts. The best practices for an integrated management are reached through the articulation of activities and fluid relations between disciplines, professions, departments, institutions, and organizations In Chile, it is the alternative to correct the inequities of the prevailing neoliberal economic model and achieve progress in the reproductive experiences of vulnerable women and families. It is a matter of justice and social responsibility. The proposed interventions contribute to the social construction of learning skills for the practice of integrated and participatory work in primary health care, where the complexity of the phenomena must be approached holistically.

Conflict of interest

The author declares no conflict of interest.

Author details

Estela Arcos Griffiths
External Researcher of the CSOC 10 18-19 Project Sponsored by the Universidad Playa Ancha, Chile

*Address all correspondence to: estelaarcos2014@gmail.com

References

[1] Braveman P, Gruskin S. Defining equity in health. J Epidemiol Community Health. 2003;57:254-258. DOI: 10.1136/jech.57.4.254

[2] Braveman P. Social conditions, health equity, and human rights. Health an Humand Rights. 2010;12(2):31-48. https://www.jstor.org/stable/healhumarigh.12.2.31

[3] Ndiaye K, KriegerJ, Warren J, Hecht M, Okuyemi K. Health Disparities and Discrimination: Three Perspectives. J Health Dispar Res Pract. 2008;2(3): 51-71. DOI: 10.1901/jaba.2008.2-51

[4] Small R, Taft A, Brown S. The power of social connection and support in improving health: lessons from social support interventions with childbearing women. BMC public health. 2011;11: S54. DOI.org/10.1186/1471-2458-11-S5-S4

[5] Alazraqui M, Mota E, Spinelli H. El abordaje epidemiológico de las desigualdades en salud a nivel local. Cad. Saúde Pública. 2007;23(2):321-330. http://dx.doi.org/10.1590/S0102-311X2007000200008

[6] Puyol Á. Ethics, equity and social determinants of health. Gac Sanit. 2012; 26(2):178-181. http://scielo.isciii.es/scielo.php?script=sci_arttext&pid=S0213-91112012000200016&lng=es.

[7] Diaz A. Economía política de la desigualad social, el reto del siglo XXI: reducir la desigualdad social. In: Economía política de la desigualad social Santo Domingo, editors, Rep. Dominicana. 2018. 326 p. https://www.researchgate.net/publication/344119510

[8] Araujo K. La calle y las desigualdades interaccionales. Serie Documentos de Trabajo PNUD–Desigualdad 2016;6:1-59. https://www.cl.undp.org/content/chile/es/home/library/poverty/documentos_de_trabajo/la-calle-y-las-desigualdades-interaccionales.html

[9] Baru RV, Mohan M. Globalisation and neoliberalism as structural drivers of health inequities. Health research policy and systems. 2018;16(Suppl1):91. DOI:10.1186/s12961-018-0365-2.

[10] Engelgau MM, Zhang P, Jan S, Mahal A. Economic Dimensions of Health Inequities: The Role of Implementation Research. Ethnicity & disease. 2019;29(Suppl 1):103-112. DOI:10.18865/ed.29.S1.103

[11] Conceição P. Más allá del ingreso, más allá de los promedios, más allá del presente. Desigualdades del Desarrollo Humano en el siglo XXI. Informe sobre desarrollo humano. Programas de las Naciones Unidas para el Desarrollo Humano (PNUD) 2019. http://hdr.undp.org/sites/default/files/hdr_2019_overview_-_spanish.pdf

[12] Venkatapuram S, Bell R, Marmot M. The right to sutures: social epidemiology, human rights, and social justice. Health and Human Rights [Internet]. 2010; 12(2):3-16. https://www.ncbi.nlm.nih.gov/pmc/articles/PMC3694312/

[13] Dulin M, Tapp H, Smith H, de Hernandez B, Coffman M, Furuseth O, et al. A trans-disciplinary approach to the evaluation of social determinants of health in a Hispanic population. BMC Public Health. 2012;12:769. https://doi.org/10.1186/1471-2458-12-769

[14] Frei R. La economía moral de la desigualdad en Chile: Un modelo para armar. Serie Documentos de trabajo. PNUD–Area Pobreza y Desigualdad. 2016/08,39p. https://www.cl.undp.org/content/chile/es/home/library/poverty/documentos_de_trabajo/

la-economia-moral-de-la-desigualdad-en-chile.html

[15] UNDP. The next frontier. Human development and the Anthropocene. Human Development Report. e United Nations Development Programme UNDP 2020, 412p. http://hdr.undp.org/sites/default/files/hdr2020.pdf

[16] OECD. In It Together: Why Less Inequality Benefits All. 2015. https://doi.org/10.1787/9789264235120-en

[17] Kmietowicz Z. Gender equality: countries are failing to deliver changes by 2030. BMJ 2019;365:l4049. DOI: https://doi.org/10.1136/bmj.l4049

[18] Basu R.L. Poverty Removal Measures of Amartya Sen and the Smithian Dilemma. Revista Científica Arbitrada de la Fundación MenteClara. 2020; 5 (115). DOI: doi.org/10.32351/rca.v5.115

[19] OECD. Gender Equality in the Pacific Alliance. Promoting Women's Economic Empowerment. OCDE Publishing, Paris. 2016. https://doi.org/10.1787/9789264262959-en

[20] Nielsen F. Inequality and inequity. Social Science Research. 2017;62:29-35. https://doi.org/10.1016/j.ssresearch.2016.12.009

[21] Sreenivasan G. Ethics and Epidemiology: Residual Health inequalities. Public Health Ethics 2009;2(3):244-249. https://doi.org/10.1093/phe/php030

[22] Gutiérrez JP, Leyva Flores R, & Aracena Genao B. Social inequality in sexual and reproductive health in Ecuador: an analysis of gaps by levels of provincial poverty 2009-2015. International Journal for Equity in Health. 2019;18(49). https://doi.org/10.1186/s12939-019-0951-0

[23] Braveman P, Gottlied G. The Social Determinants of Health: It's Time to Consider the Causes of the Causes. Public Health Reports. 2014;129(1) S1. https://doi.org/10.1177/00333549141291S206

[24] Mota, C. S., Atkin, K., Trad, L. A., & Dias A. Social disparities producing health inequities and shaping sickle cell disorder in Brazil. Health Sociology Review. 2017; 26(3), 280-292. https://doi.org/10.1080/14461242.2017.1361855

[25] Oberman, M. Motherhood, Abortion, and the Medicalization of Poverty. The Journal of Law, Medicine & Ethics : A Journal of the American Society of Law, Medicine & Ethics. 2018; 46(3):665-671. https://doi.org/10.1177/1073110518804221

[26] Kickbusch I. The political determinants of health—10 years on. BMJ 2015; 350 :h81. DOI: https://doi.org/10.1136/bmj.h81

[27] Keene D, & Padilla M. Spatial stigma and health inequality. Critical Public Health. 2014; 24(4): 392-404. https://doi.org/10.1080/09581596.2013.873532

[28] Oliver A, Healey A, & Le Grand J. Addressing health inequalities. Lancet. 2002; 360 (9332): 565-567. DOI: https://doi.org/10.1016/S0140-6736(02)09713-1

[29] Aguilera X, Delgado I, Icaza G, Apablaza M, Villanueva L, Castillo-Laborde C. Under five and infant mortality in Chile (1990-2016): Trends, disparities, and causes of death. Plos One. 2020;15(9):pp. e0239974. DOI: 10.1371/journal.pone.0239974

[30] Hensher M, Zywert K. Can healthcare adapt to a world of tightening ecological constraints? Challenges on the road to a post-growth future. BMJ. 2020; 371: m4168. DOI: https://doi.org/10.1136/bmj.m4168

[31] Cuberes D, Teignier M. Gender inequality and economic growth.

Background Paper for World Development Report 2012: Gender Equality and Development. The World Bank, Washington, DC. https://openknowledge.worldbank.org/bitstream/handle/10986/9117/WDR2012-0019.pdf?sequence=1

[32] Galvez T. Aspectos económicos de la equidad de género. Naciones Unidas, Comisión Economica para America Latina y El Caribe (CEPAL). Serie Mujer y Desarrollo. 2001 N° 35. Santiago de Chile. CEPAL Unidad Mujer y Desarrollo. https://repositorio.cepal.org/bitstream/handle/11362/5882/1/S01060530_es.pdf http://www.eclac.cl/publicaciones/UnidadMujer/1/LCL1561/lcl1561e.pdf

[33] Buvinic M, O'Donnell M. Gender Matters in Economic Empowerment Interventions: A Research Review. The World Bank Research Observer. 2019; 34 (2): 309-346. https://doi.org/10.1093/wbro/lky004.

[34] Dibaba, Y., Fantahun, M. & Hindin, M.J. The association of unwanted pregnancy and social support with depressive symptoms in pregnancy: evidence from rural Southwestern Ethiopia. BMC Pregnancy Childbirth 13, 135 (2013). https://doi.org/10.1186/1471-2393-13-135

[35] Bernazzani O, Bifulco A. Motherhood as a vulnerability factor in major depression: the role of negative pregnancy experiences. Social Science & Medicine. 2003; 56 (6): 1249-1260. https://doi.org/10.1016/S0277-9536(02)00123-5

[36] Aiser A, Currie J. The intergenerational transmission of inequality: Maternal disadvantage and health at birth. Science 2014; 344: 856-861. DOI: 10.1126/science.1251872

[37] Muñoz LA, Sánchez X, Arcos E, Vollrath A & Bonatti C. The motherhood experience in the context of social vulnerability: a comprehensive approach to social phenomenology1. Rev Latino-Am. Enfermagem. 2013; 21(4), 913-919. https://dx.doi.org/10.1590/S0104-11692013000400012

[38] Arcos E, Muñoz LA, Sánchez X, Vollrath A, Latorre C, Bonatti C et al. Vulnerabilidad social en mujeres embarazadas de una comuna de la Región Metropolitana. Rev méd. Chile 2011, 139(6),739-747. https://dx.doi.org/10.4067/S0034-98872011000600007

[39] Arcos, Estela, Canales, Mónica, Muñoz, Luz Angélica, Toffoletto, María Cecilia, Sánchez, Ximena, & Vollrath, Antonia. (2016). Invisibility of social vulnerability and social rights to a comprehensive health care in Chile. Texto & Contexto - Enfermagem, 2016;25(4),e6150015. https://dx.doi.org/10.1590/0104-07072016006150015

[40] Blake VK, McGowan ML. Filling a Federal Void: Promises and Perils of State Law in Addressing Women's Health Disparities. Journal of Law, Medicine & Ethics. 2020;48(3):485-90. DOI:10.1177/1073110520958873.

[41] Mattar L, Dinis C. Hieraquias reproductivas: Maternidade e desigualdades no exercício de direitos humanos pelas mulheres. Interface (Botucatu). 2012;16(40): 107-20. https://doi.org/10.1590/S1414-32832012005000001.

[42] Daoud N, Urquia ML, O'Campo P, Heaman M, Janssen PA, Smylie J et al. Prevalence of Abuse and Violence Before, During, and After Pregnancy in a National Sample of Canadian Women. AJPH. 2012;102(10):1893-1901. https://doi.org/10.2105/AJPH.2012.300843

[43] Zheng B, Zhu X, Hu Z, Zhou W, Yu Y, Yin S et al. The prevalence of domestic violence and its association with family factors: a cross-sectional study among pregnant women in

urban communities of Hengyang City, China. BMC Public Health. 2020;20(1):1-9. https://doi.org/10.1186/s12889-020-08683-9.

[44] Sarkar N. The impact of intimate partner violence on women's reproductive health and pregnancy outcome. Journal of Obstetrics and Gynaecology. 2008;28(3):266-271. DOI: 10.1080/01443610802042415

[45] Mauri E, Nespoli A, Persico G, & Zobbi VF. Domestic violence during pregnancy: Midwives' experiences. Midwifery. 2015; 31(5):498-504. https://doi.org/10.1016/j.midw.2015.02.002

[46] Bahadir-Yilma E & Küçük E. Unplanned and Risk Pregnancy, Domestic Violence and the Psychosocial Health Status of Pregnant Women in North-East Turkey. IJCS. 2015;8(3):585-593. http://www.internationaljournalofcaring sciences.org/

[47] Finnbogadóttir H, Dykes A, Wann-Hansson C. Prevalence of domestic violence during pregnancy and related risk factors: a cross-sectional study in southern Sweden. BMC Women's Health. 2014;14,63. https://doi.org/10.1186/1472-6874-14-63

[48] Arcos E, Uarac M, Molina I, Repossi A, Ulloa M. Impact of domestic violence on reproductive and neonatal health. Rev. méd. Chile. 2001;129(12):1413-1424. https://dx.doi.org/10.4067/S0034-98872001001200007

[49] McKeating A, Crosby D, Collins M, O'Higgins A, McMahon L, Turner M. A longitudinal study of unplanned pregnancy in a maternity hospital setting. International Journal of Gynecology and Obstetrics. 2015;128:106-109. https://doi.org/10.1016/j.ijgo.2014.08.012

[50] Horvath S, Schreiber C & Schreiber C A. Unintended Pregnancy, Induced Abortion, and Mental Health. Current Psychiatry Reports. 2017;19(11):1-6. https://doi.org/10.1007/s11920-017-0832-4

[51] Bearak J, Popinchalk A, GanatraB, Moller A-B, Tunçalp Ö, Beavin C et al. Unintended pregnancy and abortion by income, region, and the legal status of abortion: estimates from a comprehensive model for 1990-2019. Lancet Glob Health. 2020;8:e1152-61. https://doi.org/10.1016/S2214-109X(20)30315-6

[52] Casillas A, Bodenmann P, Epiney M, Ge'taz L, Irion O, Gaspoz JM et al. The Border of Reproductive Control: Undocumented immigration as a risk factor for unintended pregnancy in Switzerland. J Immigrant Minority Health. 2015;17:527-534. DOI 10.1007/s10903-013-9939-9.

[53] Lifflander A, Gaydos LMD, Hogue CJR. Circumstances of pregnancy: low Income women in Georgia describe the difference between planned and unplanned pregnancies. Maternal & Child Health Journal. 2007;11(1):81-89. doi:10.1007/s10995-006-0138-3

[54] Ministerio de Salud de Chile. Departamento de Estadística e Información de Salud. 2015: http://extranet.deis.cl/?page_id=5939

[55] Finer L, Zolna M. Unintended pregnancy in the United States: incidence and disparities, 2006. Contraception. 2011;(84):478-485. https://doi.org/10.1016/j.contraception.2011.07.013

[56] Coelho E, Andrade M, Vitoriano L, Souza J, Silva D, Gusmão M et al. Association between unplanned pregnancy and the socioeconomic context of women in the area of family health. Acta paul. enferm. 2012; 25(3): 415-422. http://dx.doi.org/10.1590/S0103-21002012000300015

[57] Quelopana A, Alcalde C. Exploring Knowledge, Belief and Experiences in Sexual and Reproductive Health in Immigrant Hispanic Women. J Immigrant Minority Health. 2014; 16:1001-1006. DOI 10.1007/s10903-013-9807-7

[58] Ayoola A. Late Recognition of Unintended Pregnancies. Public Health Nurs. 2015;32(5):462-470. DOI: 0.1111/phn.12182

[59] Yanikkerem E, Ay S, Piro N. Planned and unplanned pregnancy: Effects on health practice and depression during pregnancy. J Obstet Gynaecol Res. 2013;39(1):180-187. DOI: 10.1111/j.1447-0756.2012.01958.

[60] Kita S, Minatani M, Hikita N, Matsuzaki M, Shiraishi M, Haruna M. A Systematic Review of the Physical, Mental, Social, and Economic Problems of Immigrant Women in the Perinatal Period in Japan. J Immigrant Minority Health. 2015; 17:1863-1881. DOI 10.1007/s10903-015-0192-2

[61] Munro K, Jarvis C, Munoz M, D'Souza V, Graves L. Undocumented Pregnant Women: What Does the Literature Tell Us? J Immigrant Minority Health. 2013; 15:281-291 DOI: 10.1007/s10903-012-9587-5

[62] Uriguen García A, González J, Espinoza J, Hidalgo T, García F, Gallegos M et al. Embarazo en la adolescencia: ¿La nueva "epidemia" de los países en desarrollo? Archivos Venezolanos de Farmacologia y Terapeutica. 2019;38(3):232-245.

[63] Faisal-Cury A, Tabb K, Niciunovas G, Cunningham C, Menezes R & Huang, H. Lower education among low-income Brazilian adolescent females is associated with planned pregnancies. International Journal of Women's Health. 2017;9:43-48. DOI:10.2147/IJWH.S118911.

[64] Lewis C, Faulkner M, Scarborough, M, & Berkeley B. Preventing subsequent births for low-income adolescent mothers: an exploratory investigation of mediating factors in intensive case management. AJPH. 2012;102(10):1862-1865. DOI:10.2105/AJPH.2012.300914

[65] Sentell T, Câmara SMA, Ylli A, Velez M, Domingues MR, Bassani DG, et al. Data gaps in adolescent fertility surveillance in middle-income countries in Latin America and South Eastern Europe: Barriers to evidence-based health promotion. South Eastern European Journal of Public Health (SEEJPH).2019. DOi: 10.4119/seejph-1885.

[66] González E, Molina T. Características de la maternidad adolescente de madres a hijas. Rev. chil. obstet. ginecol. 2007;72(6):374-382. DOI 10.4067/S0717-75262007000600004

[67] Agostini C, Brown P, & Roman A. Estimando Indigencia y Pobreza Indígena Regional con Datos Censales y Encuestas de Hogares. Cuad. econ. 2010:47(135)125-150. https://dx.doi.org/10.4067/S0717-68212010000100005

[68] Arcos E, Molina I, Quezada C. Equidad en salud reproductiva en mujeres Mapuches. Sexualidad, Salud y Sociedad - Revista Latinoamericana. 2010;5:97-118. https://www.redalyc.org/articulo.oa?id=293323015006

[69] Rojas F. Pobreza y mortalidad perinatal en la población mapuche de la Araucanía. Rev. chil. pediatr. 2011;82(2):93-104. DOI:10.4067/S0370-41062011000200003

[70] Cambronero-Saiz B. Gender policies and advertising and marketing practices that affect women's health. Global Health Action. 2013;6(1):1-6. DOI:10.3402/gha.v6i0.20372

[71] Castro F, Edivey B, Peñaranda Correa F. Understanding the meanings of motherhood: the case of a prenatal care program in a health center in Popayán, Colombia. Salud Colectiva. 2011;7(3):333-45. http://www.scielo.org.ar/scielo.php?script=sci_arttext&pid=S1851-82652011000400004&lng=es.

[72] Ospina Vanegas DP, Cristancho Gómez SM, Lafaurie Villamil MM, Rubio León DC. Humanización de los servicios reproductivos desde las experiencias de las mujeres: aportes para la reflexión. Revista Cuidarte. 2020;11(2):1-13. DOI:10.15649/cuidarte.100

[73] García-Ramírez J, Vélez-Álvarez C. Latin-American public policy regarding social determinants of health. Rev salud pública. 2013; 15 (5): 731-742. http://www.redalyc.org/articulo.oa?id=42230941007

[74] Stange K. The problem of fragmentation and the need for integrative solutions. Annals of Family Medicine. 2009; 7 (2): 100-103. DOI:10.1370/afm.971

[75] OMS. Subsanar las desigualdades en una generación: Alcanzar la equidad sanitaria actuando sobre los determinantes sociales de la salud. Resumen análitico del informe final. Organización Mundial de la Salud. 2008. https://apps.who.int/iris/handle/10665/69830

[76] Arcos E, Muñoz LA, Sánchez X, Vollrath A, Gazmuri P, Baeza M. Effectiveness of the Comprehensive Childhood Protection System for vulnerable mothers and children. Rev Latino-Am Enfermagem. 2013;21(5):1071-1079. https://dx.doi.org/10.1590/S0104-11692013000500009

[77] Gallardo K, Varas L, Gallardo M. Inequality of opportunity in health: evidence from Chile. Rev. saúde pública. 2017;51:110. https://doi.org/10.11606/S1518-8787.2017051007034

[78] Telo SV, WittRR. Sexual and Reproductive Health: Team Competences in Primary Health Care Services. Ciencia & Saude Coletiva. 2018;23(11):3481-3490. DOI:10.1590/1413-812320182311.20962016.

[79] Okafor M, Ede V, Kinuthia R, Satcher D. Explication of a Behavioral Health-Primary Care Integration Learning Collaborative and Its Quality Improvement Implications. Community Mental Health J. 2018;54(8):1109-15. DOI:10.1007/s10597-017-0230-8.

[80] Binfa L, Pantoja L, Cavada G, Labarca T, Jorquera E. Assessment Of Professional Empowerment Among Midwifery Graduates In Chile. Journal of Practical & Professional Nursing. 2020. DOI:10.24966/PPN-5681/100020

[81] Binfa L, Labarca T, Jorquera E, Cavada G. Perception of Professional Empowerment among Midwifery Graduates: School of Midwifery, University of Chile. J Midwifery Women's Health. 2017;62(5):631-632. https://doi.org/10.1111/jmwh.12690

[82] Terry AL, Brown JB, Van Hoorn R, Stewart M. Evolution and 15-year effect of a pan-Canadian training program: Transdisciplinary Understanding and Training on Research-Primary Health Care. Can Fam Physician 2018;64(6):475-6. http://www.cfp.ca/content/64/6/475/tab-article-info

[83] Druetz T. Integrated primary health care in low- and middle-income countries: a double challenge. BMC medical ethics. 2018;19(Suppl 1):48. DOI:10.1186/s12910-018-0288-z.

[84] Arcos E, Poblete J, Molina I, Miranda C, Zúñiga Y, Fecci E et al.

Gender perspective in health care teaching: A pending task. Rev. méd. chil. 2007;135(6):708-717. http://dx.doi.org/10.4067/S0034-98872007000600004

[85] Gehlert S, Murray A, Sohmer D, McClintock M, Conzen S, Olopade O. The Importance of Transdisciplinary Collaborations for Understanding and Resolving Health Disparities. Social Work in Public Health. 2010;25(3/4):408-22. DOI:10.1080/19371910903241124.

[86] Stewart M, Wuite S, Ramsden V, Burge F, Beaulieu M-D, Fortin M et al. Transdisciplinary understandings and training on research: successfully building research capacity in primary health care. Can Fam Physician. 2014;60(6):581-2. PMCID: PMC4055331